MW01519437

FAA
Medical
Certification

GUIDELINES FOR PILOTS

Third Edition

250101

Richard O. Reinhart, MD
SENIOR FAA AVIATION MEDICAL EXAMINER
USAF FLIGHT SURGEON (RETIRED)

Iowa State University Press / Ames

Richard O. Reinhart, MD, is a Senior FAA Aviation Medical Examiner, retired USAF Flight Surgeon, Minnesota Air National Guard, and President of Human Factors Resources, Inc., Minneapolis, Minnesota.

© 1997, 1992 Iowa State University Press, Ames, Iowa 50014

© 1989, Richard O. Reinhart, MD, under the title *The Pilot's Medical Manual of Certification and Health Maintenance* (Future Aviation Professionals of America, special limited edition, 1989)
© 1982, Richard O. Reinhart, MD, under the title *The Pilot's Manual of Medical Certification and Health Maintenance* (Specialty Press, 1982)

⊚ Printed on acid-free paper in the United States of America

Second edition, 1992
    Through three printings
Third edition, 1997

Library of Congress Cataloging-in-Publication Data

Reinhart, Richard O.
FAA medical certification : guidelines for pilots / Richard O. Reinhart.—3rd ed.
p.   cm.
Some previous eds. published with title: The Pilot's manual of medical certification and health maintenance.
Include bibliographical references and index.
ISBN 0-8138-2769-8
1. Air pilots—Medical examinations.   2. Air pilots—Health and hygiene.
I. Title.
RC1063.R44   1997
616.9'80213—dc21   97-18886

Last digit is the print number: 9 8 7 6 5 4 3 2 1

Contents

Foreword

Nothing seems more threatening to a pilot than the fear of losing FAA medical certification. This fear is reinforced by misperceptions of the intent of aeromedical standards and by the inherent complexity of bureaucracy. Most pilots and many doctors do not fully understand the unique physiological requirements of flight and can be misled into thinking that the standards are too restrictive.

In reality, few medical conditions are not ultimately certifiable, but the pilot is obligated to prove to the FAA that his or her medical disorder is an acceptable risk in flight. If you are fit to fly and will remain so in flight and the near future, you should be medically certified. For example, of the total number of applications received, the overall denial rate is less than 0.7 percent. Of these denials, over 50 percent failed to provide the information needed by the FAA or did not pursue the recertification process.

In my thirty-year experience as the FAA manager of Aeromedical Certification, we were able to use current technologies and aeromedical insights to certify many pilots who only a few years earlier would not even have been considered. Yet there was (and still is) the persistent frustration to my staff of dealing with administrative errors. Sometimes half the applications had omissions, errors in entries, absence of explanation of affirmative responses to the history, and other oversights that required additional time and more information.

It should be clear, therefore, that the main problems experienced with medical certification are the results of misunderstanding of what can be certified and of inadequate preparation of files. The only solution is through education of individual pilots, ideally during initial and recurrent training. But a pilot will not usually call the FAA or the AME for advice when a medical problem is identified. Pilots go first to their instructors, check airmen, managers, and ground school instructors, so these people especially need to know what to expect.

Most of the answers and solutions are addressed in this manual on FAA medical certification. It is understandable to all, comprehensive in its coverage of issues of certification and recertification, and complete in its survey of the expectations of the FAA, the Guide for AMEs, and the medical regulations. The book's useful contents are essential to maintain medical certification—it's good insurance, and it removes the mystery of the process.

It is generally accepted that most pilots do not consider the possibility of losing their medical certification until it happens. Then there is a frantic attempt to get the right information. This form of crisis management is unnecessary if you are familiar with the process and have ready access to this manual. It should be in your personal aviation library as well as on the shelves where you work or train. FAA medical certification need not be a stressful situation, but you must take the initiative of understanding your options and responsibilities. That information is in this book.

AUDIE W. DAVIS, MD
Manager, FAA Aeromedical Certification Division (Retired)

Preface

"**P**eople who live in fear of disease are apt to become ill. Anxiety quickly demoralizes the whole body and lays it open to illness and disease." James Allen, who wrote *As a Man Thinketh* in the 1800s, describes the predicament of many pilots, both professional and recreational. They are justifiably apprehensive about how to maintain or improve their health without jeopardizing their careers or medical certificates.

As a result, the medical certification process of pilots, especially those who earn a living by flying, is an emotional, often threatening, experience. The process is misunderstood by all except by those sitting in judgment and is thought by many to create more problems than it resolves. The recent (effective September 1996) changes to FAA medical standards generated a deluge of criticisms prior to being final, with many comments indicating misinterpretations of the intent of the rules. Medical certification benefits not only the individual pilot but also the entire aviation industry and those who use it.

I find it frustrating that, with a career, an employer's investment, and the sheer joy of flying for pleasure in jeopardy, few pilots truly understand or respect health maintenance and medical certification. When suffering from an unexplained pain, a pilot is anxious that it will result in being grounded. Comrades compound this anxiety by sharing misleading "war stories" to illustrate their own interpretations of certification. The result, unfortunately, is a strong case of denial and apathy that quickly turns into crisis management whenever medical certification is challenged. It appears that only those pilots who have lost their medical certification or have it threatened want to discuss the subject, and they are, of course, angry, defensive, and confused.

To my knowledge, few books address the all-important certification process—certainly no book written for pilots by a pilot who is also a physician and an experienced FAA Aviation Medical Examiner (AME). Well-meaning articles appear in trade journals and magazines and some company and union newsletters, but I have yet to see a comprehensive, unbiased explanation of the entire certification process, including the medical standards that pilots are expected to meet. Furthermore, many companies do little to protect medical certification or to provide education about the process; instead they claim it is the pilot's responsibility. A pilot's greatest fear is a medical condition of any degree of significance being prematurely reported to the FAA. Yet little has been written on what pilots can realistically do to protect their health and medical certification. This book provides that knowledge and instructs you, the pilot, in the procedures and guidelines used by your AME and the FAA. Most importantly, the book discusses the development of a health maintenance program that will give you a head start should any medical problem develop.

This book is intended primarily for professional pilots, because they must meet the strictest medical standards and because they have the greatest responsibility in the air (and the most to lose if they don't pass the physical exam). The concepts discussed, however, are useful for any pilot who wants to maintain his or her health and medical certification. Fortunately the professional pilot has an all-important motivating factor for staying healthy—a career! No other professional person is so dependent on proving good health to a boss and to a government agency. Yet despite this motivation, it is surprising to see so many pilots who abuse their health, rationalizing that they will deal with a problem when it occurs.

The philosophy expressed here is my own and is not meant to interfere with an acceptable health maintenance program that a pilot or company may already be following. My comments and opinions are addressed to those pilots who are, or feel that they are, aeromedically neglected.

Neither is this book meant to be a dissertation on any scientific medical study. It purposely avoids many sides of a controversial subject but, at the same time, attempts to define the subject's issues for the pilot. To my colleagues in aviation medical departments who want to keep their pilots healthy and flying: I share your frustration in coping with the misunderstandings of your professional goals. The occasional opinion that flight surgeons or aviation doctors are "out to get" the pilot should have disappeared at the same time that it was realized that mechanics could fix airplanes just as well as pilots—or better. To the concerned pilot who has picked up this book: I hope I may give you some facts with which to challenge the rumors you hear. There is nothing new or unique in my program for pilots. I only hope to clarify the multitude of misconceptions concerning medical certification and health maintenance (especially with new FAA medical standards in effect). Misinformation puts you at the mercy of the AME and the FAA. However, by becoming familiar with the whole process of your medical certification, you won't need the FAA to force you to be healthy. Instead, you can keep a step ahead of the FAA by using the same medical tools that the AME and the FAA use and, as a result, actually assist your AME or private medical doctor in keeping you certified. Being in control is what you enjoy about flying. You can also take control of your medical status and medical certificate. You don't have to blindly depend on your doctor and the bureaucracy to keep you flying.

The simple objective of this book is to provide you, the pilot, with the medical and administrative tools to protect your health and your medical certificate for as long as possible. I am confident that with this added knowledge you can greatly improve your odds against being forced into early medical retirement and continuing a truly enjoyable and fulfilling activity—flying.

Introduction

Professional pilots—corporate, airline, charter, military, or instructor—have the potential to lose more by having an annual physical examination than any other professional because there is a possibility the exam will keep them from flying. Yet the person who earns a living flying airplanes is more likely to be healthy because he or she came to the profession in near-perfect health and that health has been monitored frequently.

It follows that all aviators, whether professional or general/recreational, must accept and follow the same principles. Therefore, even though the term *professional pilot* is frequently used in this book, all who wish to continue flying need to know this information.

Why do a significant percentage of professional pilots never reach retirement? How can so many "healthy" pilots be medically grounded for months and even years before being returned to flying status? With a career at stake, why do professional pilots abuse their health and fail to follow the advice of doctors and other medical experts and consultants who are trying to keep them healthy and certified?

The answers to these questions are basically simple: apathy, laziness, and ignorance—all leading to fear and mistrust. Apathy about the urgency of maintaining health, laziness or procrastination in pursuing a good health maintenance program, and ignorance or lack of understanding of their medical status and the FAA's medical certification process. Put another way, pilots have frequent contact with medical professionals and health care information, but many do not take advantage of these valuable resources. They don't know how, or—worse yet—they are afraid to ask, especially if they feel fine.

Professional pilots, like the rest of us, always fear that something serious will be found unexpectedly during an exam, especially if they have symptoms, even minimal ones. Unlike most of us, however, pilots fear that some problem will be found when they are feeling great and have no symptoms. In addition, pilots fear that even if a family doctor and AME prove they are healthy the paperwork will get screwed up somewhere in the bureaucracy—and it can. In each of these situations, not only is the pilot's health in question but his or her career is threatened.

Yet, despite potentially being grounded as a result of the annual (or semi-annual) exam, professional pilots are fortunate in terms of the support they receive for their health. As an instrument-rated commercial pilot, a retired flight surgeon for the Minnesota Air National Guard, and a practitioner and consultant of aviation medicine and aeromedical certification, I am in regular, direct contact with professional pilots and have observed the following about the health of pilots.

PILOT HEALTH CHARACTERISTICS

Professional pilots are inherently healthy. To be hired or certified by the FAA as medically fit, pilots are medically screened from many applicants, most of whom are healthier than the majority of their nonaviator friends. Therefore, before pilots even begin their careers, practically all chronic diseases are proven to be absent.

A professional pilot's health is monitored periodically to ensure continued good health. Every six or twelve months pilots must prove to the FAA (and themselves) the absence of any major illness or potentially incapacitating medical problem. (Note that the exam is not meant to determine if pilots are healthy. The intent is to rule out a future medical problem in flight.) Granted, the FAA physical is no more beneficial than the doctor giving the exam. We both know that there are exams and then there are exams, and the results can be handled in a multitude of ways. (Some results are mishandled—more on this later.) Yet the fact remains: as a pilot your regular medical evaluations put you miles and years ahead of most people.

A professional pilot has the strongest motivation to maintain health: the preservation of a career! Despite this incentive—but armed with apathy and complacency (and some unrealistic feelings of invincibility)—the typical professional pilot does one of four things regarding health and medical certification:

1. Pursues a good health maintenance program and looks for potential medical risks, consequently greatly improving the probability of retaining a medical certificate.

2. Respects and trusts the FAA examiner and seeks his or her help after any medical problem arises but does little to practice a health maintenance program. A mild variation of crisis management.

3. Chooses an FAA examiner not out of trust or respect but "because the examiner's certified me for years without any question." The pilot then seeks help from another doctor (usually not experienced in aviation medicine) for medical problems. Unfortunately, many of these doctors have little knowledge of the flying profession and how "usual and customary medical care" affects FAA medical certification, flying responsibilities, and career. Their well-intended comment of "I see no reason why you can't be certified" frequently is contrary to the FAA's medical standards for a safe pilot, but worse, it misleads the pilot and begins a nightmare of conflicting medical opinions.

4. Merely gets by the FAA exam (with fingers crossed) and waits out the

next six months hoping nothing develops. This is especially common among older pilots who feel secure in their jobs and younger pilots who feel medically invincible. The philosophy is to worry about a medical grounding only if and when it happens. In other words, the idea is to avoid making waves—these pilots will worry about their health when they retire. This is a major variation of crisis management.

A professional pilot has the time and the money to pursue a worthwhile health maintenance program. The FAA exam is not usually adequate for monitoring a pilot's health. To be beneficial, a medical evaluation needs to be comprehensive with subsequent correction of current and potential problems and assistance in teaching basic medical principles. However, most of the time and money in anyone's budget is not put to medical use until a tangible and immediate need arises. Often there seem to be higher-priority needs for the pilot's time and money—until that pilot is grounded. Then there is no limit to the measures a pilot will pursue to unravel this dilemma. This predicament invariably occurs years after the medical problem could have been resolved or prevented. Most professional pilots really need to sit back and say, "Hey, I'm not as healthy as I could be. My career isn't that secure, and my loss-of-license insurance isn't the answer if I develop a medical problem." Time and money spent on health maintenance now are the best ways to secure your future.

Professional pilots have vast resources with which to educate themselves in health maintenance. Most professional pilots are well informed, but they are not physicians or flight doctors. Much of their medical information, therefore, is found in the lay press, which relates to the general population. The advice usually does not consider the unique and restrictive medical criteria to which a professional pilot must adhere to be fit to fly; consequently this general advice is of questionable usefulness. To add to the confusion, there are conflicting professional viewpoints within the health profession on very basic and fundamental health habits. Yet pilots are continually reading and exchanging new thoughts among themselves about nutrition, physical conditioning, and health maintenance. How much of this sometimes overwhelming information is beneficial and understood—and how to apply it—is another matter. For health education, prudent pilots can and should turn to their flight physicians for information, just as they would turn to aircraft mechanics for airplane maintenance.

Some professional pilots can depend on an organization or union for assistance when medical trouble develops or medical certification is lost. Such support by a peer organization or company medical department often reinforces apathy and a false sense of security. Valuable as these groups may be in restoring certification, they are already behind the wall of red tape, an obstacle that must be overcome even before they can start to resolve the pilot's individual difficulty. Much credit is due their efforts, but I'm sure that an all too common feeling is "if only I had done something to prevent or find this problem earlier." *If only* are two mighty small words when it comes to restoring your medical certification. Ultimately, with or without organizational support, the pilot is still fighting this battle alone.

Professional pilots have "clout," enabling them to change their working environment, to improve their performance, and to preserve their medical flying status. Flying people in "friendly skies" is a major responsibility for pilot and management. It is unlikely that either side would irresponsibly ignore legitimate suggestions for improving the achievement of this basic goal of keeping aircraft and pilots flying safely. However, the intent of a change can be misinterpreted or get bogged down in petty bureaucratic and personal goals, budgetary constraints, and contractual conditions so that the objective is lost in the shuffle. The result in the aviation business, unfortunately, is sometimes a defensive attitude by management, the FAA, or the pilot group, whereby this clout is used negatively as a weapon or bargaining tool.

From the foregoing it is clear that pilots do, in fact, have more control over their medical destiny than they might realize or be willing to accept—providing they can cope with those who will be judging them and maintain patience with the complex system of meeting medical standards.

So what to do? You are one against that system, with a career at stake, required to work with complex and frequently misunderstood aeromedical rules and regulations. Recent 1996 changes do much to clarify previous misconceptions and have made standards more realistic. Your medical status is not understood by some nonaviation doctors who are misinformed about FAA protocol and can lead you into the FAA's red tape. And you expect that if you are not healthy, you will be reported immediately to the FAA and grounded. Yet you have the best odds of staying healthy and certified if you are willing to accept the responsibility of controlling your medical status.

There are many factors you alone can control for your benefit as an aviator to better the odds of maintaining satisfactory health for yourself, your employer, and the FAA. There are no magic solutions—though the means are simple and basic. I do not attempt to imply that any health maintenance program will guarantee you a flying career until you choose to retire. I do, however, guide you through a program that is realistic, factual, and adaptable to your specific responsibilities, and I try to provide a clearer picture of old and new FAA medical standards and policies.

You do have control over your medical future, flying career, and your desire to keep flying! Take control *now*—don't wait to reach for the stick after things start falling apart!

FAA Medical Certification

1

The Philosophy of Pilot Health Monitoring and Health Maintenance

You're at lunch before a turn-around trip ...

"Hey George, what do you think? My family doc gave me some pills to take because he said my blood pressure is up a bit. I don't think he knows I'm a pilot. What should I do?"

George: "Don't sweat it, Fred. Just don't say anything at your FAA exam and hope your blood pressure is OK."

Or over a beer at the end of a trip ...

"Jack, I've been meaning to ask you ... I took an insurance exam and they said there was something wrong with my urine. My FAA physical is due next month. What the hell should I do?"

Jack: "No problem, Fred. See my examiner. He never checks my urine and, in fact, really doesn't do much at all. That's why I see him. Why rock the boat, right?"

Why look for a problem when you're feeling fine? Why not wait until something goes wrong and then tell the family doctor? Why say anything to the FAA if you think you're OK? And how is it going to find out anyway? This is the way the majority of pilots reason when discussing their medical certification.

But when it comes to your airplane, you have a different set of values and priorities. Don't you actively seek out a problem or potential malfunction even if you know the bird is flying well? You preflight, you follow checklists, you subject your flying machine to periodic exams. Next to maintaining your flying proficiency, you are most possessive about maintaining the airworthiness of the aircraft you fly.

FAA'S HEALTH-MONITORING PROGRAM

There is a valid reason for the FAA health-monitoring program. However, fear and skepticism about the FAA and its medical exams come from misunderstanding the medical certification process and the impact of some medical problems on flying safely. A comparison of the periodic maintenance inspection of your aircraft with the practice of health maintenance will clarify the importance of your required FAA medical exam.

It seems to me that your "human machine" deserves no less concern and maintenance than your flying machine. I am certain that all responsible pilots would welcome the resources with which to provide themselves the same level of maintenance of their health as they expect will be provided for their aircraft. Why doesn't it happen? Because they fear losing their medical certification and career once their questionable health status is reported to the FAA.

Pilots wouldn't fly if they knew they had a problem that would suddenly incapacitate them or create a distraction on the flight deck. An approach to minimums in turbulence is not the time to have your buddy cry out in pain or faint! Contrary to popular belief, and medically speaking, your company, your doctors, and the FAA have only one goal regarding your medical status: to keep you healthy and free of disabling or distracting medical problems—to keep you fit to fly and flying safely. Is that any different than your personal philosophy on the responsibilities of piloting? There shouldn't be two standards.

Now that we agree on this basic philosophy, let's rush to our FAA examiner and say, "Hey Doc, see if I've got any problem that is going to make me unsafe to fly." Why the chuckles? Did I hear somebody say, "No way"? Obviously, in spite of all of our well-intentioned objectives, the environment that would encourage pilots to seek their personal "preventive maintenance" just doesn't exist.

Why not?

It's difficult, if not impossible, to explain to each pilot's satisfaction the purpose of health monitoring for a pilot who feels fine: "How can I have a disqualifying problem if I don't feel sick? Besides, I know plenty of pilots in worse shape, and nobody questions them." Pilots are challenged by well-established contradictions, misconceptions, historically poor medical evaluations and follow-ups, plus "testimonials" that would discredit most attempts to justify even the best intentions of FAA examiners, family doctors, and flight surgeons. And the aviation press does little to provide unbiased reasoning for FAA medical standards. Just recall the furor within the press concerning the age sixty rule, the new medical standards, and drug and alcohol testing. So what to do?

Let's start at the beginning. I believe we can make one fundamental statement of fact. Everyone, especially you, wants the crew of your aircraft (and that includes you) to be free of any medical deficiency that would interfere with safely and competently flying a machine from point A to point B. The pilot, however, wants this to be done without risking being booted out of flying for a living. There's the contradiction. But I can assure you that if pilots do their part in learning the principles of health maintenance and how the FAA certifies them, there need not be the unnecessary threat that all pilots feel when their health is discussed or evaluated.

Pilots, like the rest of society, rely heavily on rules and regulation, company policies, standards, and SOPs to guide and direct them. If something does go wrong, they often can pass the buck to the rule maker or enforcer and thereby relieve themselves of the responsibility. Not so with the pilot's health and medical certificate. The buck stops with the pilot! You are the one held accountable for being fit to fly.

Pilots already have been educated to ensure that their airplanes meet mechanical and electronic criteria with the necessary help of specialists and engineers. In this regard, we have an enviable team. Yet, being human, we have a tendency to take shortcuts or to forget pertinent data in this complex profession, which is why we have checklists and proficiency checks. Also, as in any field of work, someone periodically has to check up on, or monitor, what we are doing. This is a fact of life—no venture can meet the expectations of the people it services without some sort of monitoring. Otherwise, chaos would rule, and the few who abuse the rules will set their own standards. So all of us need and silently expect someone to respectfully say, "Hey, what you're doing is OK," or "What you're doing isn't OK and you need to improve." Or, "Were you aware that what you are doing is in violation of the rules?" This is true of pilots, as we all know. It is also true of businesspeople, teachers, lawyers, and, believe it or not, doctors.

How many times have you been to your private physician and felt you did not receive the best service that medicine could provide? As a doctor, I'm the first to say that you could, in fact, have been denied the best. Patients deserve the assurance of competent help, just as your passengers expect you, unconditionally, to do your job safely—they expect a routine, uneventful flight each trip. What goes on behind that cockpit door is your business—as long as you do it right. To ensure this, you must be monitored, even though you feel fine and you think you're healthy. Whose responsibility is this monitoring? Your peers protect you with professional standards and aeromedical committees. Your company protects you and its shareholders with check rides, company physicals, operating policies, and insurance. And the FAA is mandated to protect the public from medically unsafe pilots through Federal Air Regulations and medical certification. The 1996 changes to the medical regulations, the first for many years, have made the evaluation process more realistic, flexible, and understandable.

With the FAA's involvement in this monitoring process, a multitude of things can happen—which is why the acronym *FAA* conjures up a vision of a many-headed monster armed with a protocol on how to shaft the aviator at every turn. However, it is important to understand the FAA's health-monitoring philosophy and to realize what you can do to keep the bureaucratic monster happy.

Let's review what I've stated so far:

1. Responsible pilots do not want to fly if they know their health is going to interfere with their flying ability or potentially cause a disaster, and they certainly don't want anyone else flying in poor health.

2. There must be a monitoring program to protect, guide, and assist the pilot and the pilot's peers, employer, and passengers.

3. The FAA has been delegated as the government's agency to provide this monitoring program on behalf of the public.

4. The new medical standards take into account current medical insights along with experience on what standards are effective.

THE ROLE OF PILOT AND AVIATION EXAMINER IN THE FAA'S PROGRAM

At the point of the FAA medical exam, the process of ensuring that only healthy pilots are flying often breaks down. Again, contrary to popular belief, the intent of the FAA is not to ground pilots for insignificant medical reasons. The process will be discussed later, but for now let's make our first assumption.

Let's assume the FAA's sole medical goal is to ensure that pilots do not have a medical problem that would create an unsafe situation. This means that the FAA wants a pilot fit to fly at the time of the exam and for six to twelve months afterward. It's senseless to assume otherwise. (I am not discussing the age sixty rule.) No one wants a pilot to become impaired in flight. It is also a fair assumption that most aircrews have little, if any, medical training, compared with the extent of their education about the aircraft, its components, and the environment in which they fly. It is ironic and unfortunate that of the two most important parts of air travel, the pilot and the machine, the pilot is well educated only in the mechanics of the airplane and not in the mechanics of his or her health and special medical maintenance requirements as a pilot. If some pilots treated their aircraft the way they treat their bodies, they would never reach their destination.

The military recognizes this need and quite effectively uses the "flight surgeon" system, which requires that all flying personnel must see only a flight surgeon for all medical care—therapy, examination, general health care, and certification of flying status. The flight surgeon is specifically trained in aviation medicine and devotes full time to it, a fact that is generally recognized and respected by the aircrews. The result is trust and mutual understanding and good medical care if the flight surgeon is reliable. And pilots are flying when they are healthy! The flight surgeon has the authority to return a pilot to flying status immediately.

The military flight surgeon's civilian counterpart, the FAA-designated Aviation Medical Examiner (AME), is not required to be specifically trained in aviation medicine beyond a three-day "familiarization course" and periodic refreshers. AMEs may devote most of their time to the practice of nonaviation medicine (they may be family doctors, surgeons, or other specialists) and fit pilots in as their schedule permits. Just being a doctor does not ensure adequate knowledge of a specific subject, such as aviation medicine and aeromedical certification.

Another vitally important difference is that the military flight surgeon is considered to be a part of the crew he or she serves. The flight surgeon flies with, encounters delays with, eats questionable meals with, and suffers long days and short nights with the rest of the crew. The flight surgeon develops an acquaintance with the crew's peculiar physical and mental stresses and gets to know pilot teammates individually. The crew also gets the chance to see just what the flight surgeon is up to and can check him or her out, seeing whose side the flight surgeon is on. In the civilian aviation world, on the other hand, flying the jump seat is discouraged for even the most well-meaning AME. Furthermore, most civilian doctors and even AMEs are more interested in pilots' clinical status than in the essentially nonchallenging aspect of medical certification.

To a certain extent the FAA attempts to follow the philosophy of the military flight surgeon system. The Federal Air Surgeon in Washington, D.C., has overall responsibility for aviation medicine and its consequences. The primary responsibility of medical certification is delegated to the FAA doctors in Oklahoma City. These doctors, in turn, have designated civilian physicians throughout the country to conduct the examinations for the FAA doctors. These local doctors, or AMEs, have no authority except to certify healthy pilots— healthy as determined by the individual AME but still subject to review by the FAA's doctors. To the FAA's credit, it is allowing more authority to be granted to AMEs to certify pilots they feel are an acceptable risk, and the new medical regulations give further guidance for implementing this policy.

This process is why, for example, if your AME tells you that you have a "slight heart murmur" but does not feel it is of any consequence, the AME has no authority to certify you without approval from the FAA Regional Flight Surgeon or the FAA physician in Oklahoma City. Sometimes, since the AME doesn't want to be the "bad guy," he or she may certify you, only to have your health reviewed (or monitored) later by the FAA. Weeks later, the FAA will ask for more information and data *from you* to determine if the murmur is significant or potentially unsafe. The AME really could have done that to begin with, but for various reasons the AME has chosen to let the FAA do it. You're the one, however, whose career is on the line and, in your mind, who now is being challenged.

Another policy of some AMEs is to not even check for any potential problems. It would appear that this "planned ignorance" keeps the pilots and the AME content, but those pilots ultimately sacrifice their health to protect their careers—and often needlessly. Such rubber stamping AMEs are around; worse, they often have a large following since they are the least threatening. In theory, this is the epitome of irresponsibility, like ignoring a SIGMET or a thunderstorm simply because you have to get to your destination on time. But realistically, if I were in the same medical situation as a professional pilot with my career at stake, I would be tempted to respond the same way. By ignoring potential problems, both the pilot and the doctor can plead innocent and make the FAA accept the responsibility. However, chances are the pilot will ultimately lose.

Although the FAA doctors often are made out to be the villains, they really aren't every time. The FAA, accept it or not, is no more a threat to your health and career than some AMEs who should be acting in your best interests but, in fact, are not. Why doesn't the FAA's program of pilot health monitoring work to the benefit of the pilot as well as the FAA?

One of the prime reasons is lack of adequate education and communication. You and I are trying to correct that. If you know why certain tests are done and what is at stake, you have better control of your future. I will elaborate more on the specific protocol that is followed, why it is essential, and how you can keep control. For now, keep in mind that the greatest deterrent to the maintenance of your certification may be your peers and a few of the FAA's uninformed, inexperienced AMEs, who, by simply going through the motions and assuming they're doing you a favor, leave you holding the bag. So what should you expect in the certification process?

THE CIVILIAN FLIGHT SURGEON

It is imperative that you be under the supervision of a physician who is knowledgeable in aviation medicine, FAA criteria, and the certification process. Such an AME must act like a military flight surgeon, whose goal is to keep you flying safely. The doctor must pursue the evaluation and certification process until a satisfactory result is achieved. That means, in addition to treating you in a manner acceptable to the FAA, the doctor will coordinate, follow through, and personally ensure that your certification is not compromised, that the medical data are accurate and complete, and that you are kept informed.

The AME/Flight Surgeon should guide you in how to keep healthy to control your medical status. Together, you will monitor trends in the results of your exams and try to anticipate potential certification problems, resolving them before they interfere with your career. You should feel relatively comfortable in describing your aches, pains, and other complaints and be able to work together. After all, this doc should be a member of your team, as important to you as a mechanic or meteorologist.

Finding this perfect physician isn't all that easy, as we know. But until you do, there is the next-best thing: a health maintenance program. In your situation, that also means an "FAA certification and career maintenance" program. Remember, your AME has little or no authority to keep you flying unless you are truly healthy. The buck is still in your lap. And the regulations state so: look up FAR 61.53.

There are some things about your health that you can't control. You can't pick your parents, you can't alter your genes, and you can't change your potential for developing a disease not related to environment, such as cancer or vision changes. In these situations, loss-of-license insurance and company benefits won't cure you or keep you flying.

But there are areas you can control, factors that, ignored or abused, invariably lead to deterioration of health that will affect only a pilot's career. With so much at stake—your career and love of flying—it would seem reasonable to expect that you would do everything possible to maintain your health, not waiting for a problem to get your attention. That means preventive maintenance just like the kind you provide the airplane in which you fly. Being grounded doesn't just happen to someone else. Your grounded buddy was feeling good too before he got the ax. No one can do this work for you. No one can undo any permanent damage you have already allowed to occur, and no physician can do your health maintenance work; indeed, physicians often can create more problems by letting you avoid this work.

You are quite capable of controlling the controllable elements of your health. Quit reading about the latest fad diets and physical conditioning programs in the tabloids and the popular lay magazines and books. They are not coming up with anything that is revolutionary. You wouldn't take flying lessons from them, so don't take their aeromedical lessons either.

IN REVIEW

1. You are in a profession that requires you to be free of diseases that would interfere in the performance of your duties. "Feeling good" is not a true indicator of your health.

2. As in any other work, you must be monitored, and the FAA monitors you by using local AMEs as their tools.

3. The process of medical certification through some local doctors with

varying degrees of aeromedical knowledge, experience with the FAA, and interest in aviation often leads to ignorance concerning your actual medical status. Consequently, your health is sacrificed for the sake of your career. It needn't be that way.

4. Finding a physician you can regard as a competent, respected "flight surgeon" is difficult. All too often, pilots seek the doctor that makes the fewest waves.

5. You are not concerned so much about being sick as you are about what happens when you are reported to the FAA. However, you will have the best chance of remaining certified if you program yourself to be healthy, informed, in top physical condition, and knowledgeable about the FAA's certification process.

With the philosophy of pilot health monitoring and health maintenance in mind, let's look more closely at the medical *standards* the FAA expects you to meet.

2

Disqualifying Medical Conditions

A thirty-six-year-old airline pilot was seeing her family doctor on an annual basis in anticipation of her FAA exam. Her family doctor noted her blood pressure had gone above 140/90 and put her on a new blood pressure medication. At her next FAA exam her blood pressure was still high, plus the pilot had to report that she was on medication. Three weeks later the FAA grounded her because of the hypertension, the use of the blood pressure medication, and no medical reports.

Basically, the FAA has fair medical criteria for certification of healthy pilots. In fact, if you were aware of the reasoning behind the FAA's medical decisions, you would probably agree with the conclusions that are in most cases challenged by pilots.

Now I'm sure that many of you are skeptical as you read this, especially if your opinion is based on your experiences, those of your colleagues, and your interpretation of the FAA certification process. In defense, let me state clearly that I am in no way crusading for the FAA and its bureaucracy. I do believe, however, that the majority of medical decisions made about an individual pilot are fair, providing the FAA doctors have been given adequate documentation of that pilot's true medical status. I can appreciate your skepticism, but if you bear with me, you will understand why I make such a controversial comment.

AMENDED FAR PART 67

Before continuing, it's important to bring up how the 1996 revised Federal Air Regulation (FAR) Part 67, "Medical Standards and Certification," differs from previous editions. This is the first major review and revision in many years and was the result of a 1982 report from the American Medical Association (AMA) at the request of the FAA. The Notice for Proposed Rule Making (NPRM) was issued in October 1994 and released as a final rule in March 1996 with an effective date of September 16, 1996. During that fourteen-year period there were probably more discussions and arguments than there were over any other proposed changes! In fact, when it was known that the FAA had finalized its

Part 67 Medical Standards
Effective September 16, 1996

Medical Certificate Pilot Type	First-Class Airline Transport Pilot	Second-Class Commercial Pilot	Third- Class Private Pilot
DISTANT VISION	20/20 or better in each eye separately, with or without correction.		20/40 or better in each eye separately, with or without correction.
NEAR VISION	20/40 or better in each eye separately (Snellen equivalent), with or without correction, as measured at 16 inches.		
INTERMEDIATE VISION	20/40 or better in each eye separately (Snellen equivalent), with or without correction, at age 50 and over, as measured at 32 inches.		No requirement.
COLOR VISION	Ability to perceive those colors necessary for safe performance of airman duties.		
HEARING	Demonstrate hearing of an average conversational voice in a quiet room, using both ears at 6 feet, with the back turned to the examiner <u>or</u> pass one of the audiometric tests below.		
AUDIOLOGY	Audiometric speech discrimination test: Score at least 70 % discrimination in one ear.		
	Pure tone audiometric test: Unaided, with thresholds no worse than: <table><tr><td></td><td>500 Hz</td><td>1,000 Hz</td><td>2,000 Hz</td><td>3,000 Hz</td></tr><tr><td>Better Ear</td><td>35 Db</td><td>30 Db</td><td>30 Db</td><td>40 Db</td></tr><tr><td>Worst Ear</td><td>35 Db</td><td>50 Db</td><td>50 Db</td><td>60 Db</td></tr></table>		
ENT	No ear disease or condition manifested by, or that may reasonably be expected to be manifested by, vertigo or a disturbance of speech or equilibrium.		
PULSE	Not disqualifying, *per se*. Used to determine cardiac system status and responsiveness.		
BLOOD PRESSURE	No specified values stated in the standards. Hypertension covered under general medical standard and in the *Guide for Aviation Medical Examiners*.		
ELECTROCARDIOGRAM (ECG)	At age 35 and annually after age 40.	Not routinely required.	
MENTAL	No diagnosis of psychosis, or bipolar disorder, or severe personality disorders.		
SUBSTANCE DEPENDENCE AND SUBSTANCE ABUSE	A diagnosis or medical history of "substance dependence" is disqualifying unless there is established clinical evidence, satisfactory to the Federal Air Surgeon, of recovery, including sustained total abstinence from the substance(s) for not less than the preceding 2 years. A history of "substance abuse" within the preceding 2 years is disqualifying. "Substance" includes alcohol and other drugs (i.e., PCP, sedatives and hynoptics, anxiolytics, marijuana, cocaine, opioids, amphetamines, hallucinogens, and other psychoactive drugs or chemicals).		
DISQUALIFYING CONDITIONS* *BOLD print depicts new disqualifying conditions as of September 16, 1996. Substance dependence and abuse replace drug dependence and alcoholism.	Examiner must disqualify if the applicant has a history of: (1) Diabetes mellitus requiring hypoglycemic medication; (2) Angina pectoris; (3) Coronary heart disease that has been treated or, if untreated, that has been symptomatic or clinically significant; (4) Myocardial infarction; **(5) Cardiac valve replacement; (6) Permanent cardiac pacemaker; (7) Heart replacement**; (8) Psychosis; **(9) Bipolar disorder**; (10) Personality disorder that is severe enough to have repeatedly manifested itself by overt acts; **(11) Substance dependence; (12) Substance abuse**; (13) Epilepsy; (14) Disturbance of consciousness without satisfactory explanation of cause; and **(15) Transient loss of control of nervous system function(s) without satisfactory explanation of cause.**		

NOTE: For further information, contact your Regional Flight Surgeon (phone numbers are in Appendix C of the *Guide for Aviation Medical Examiners*).

Overview of FARs Part 67 medical standards

rule in August 1994, there was an additional administrative delay during which everyone was speculating on how disruptive the new regulation would be. The final released rule, however, was far from threatening.

A key point to remember about the old and the new standards is that the rule (FAR Part 67) is not meant to be too specific. That is, the AME and FAA still interpret an individual's medical history, examinations, and test results to determine if a pilot is a flight risk. The interpretation of the rule by the AME and FAA is assisted by the *Guide for Aviation Medical Examiners* (see Appendix II). FAR Part 67 no longer states specific quantitative requirements (such as blood pressure readings); these are defined in the guide. The guide is reviewed in Appendix II and is meant only to define some of the terminology and intent of FAR Part 67's standards and is not meant to be definitive in establishing the certifiability of a specific medical problem. That's where your AME comes in, and that will be discussed later.

In fact, I discourage you from seeking too much information about your individual situation solely by reviewing FAR Part 67, the guide, and this manual. Don't play doctor or AME. There are obviously subtle differences between one person and another with the same disorder, and they can't be comprehensively explained by a book.

MEDICAL SPECIFICATIONS

Having said that, I would like to return to the analogy of the preventive maintenance program for your aircraft. There are tech orders, books on specifications, operation standards, ADs, and a multitude of other complex, specific criteria that must be met during each periodic preventive maintenance inspection of the aircraft. A mechanic may simply sign off on an aircraft and by so doing tell you that the craft is airworthy and safe, but you have the right and the responsibility to check the records and the aircraft to ensure that all of the specifications have, in fact, been met. You are not second-guessing the mechanic. In fact, most responsible mechanics are proud of their job and welcome the pilot's interest in their work. And you both speak the same language because, during your initial and recurrent training, you have been educated as to how these specs were determined, why they are important, and what restrictions must be met. In other words, you know what keeps your machine flying.

Meeting certain detailed specifications is no different when it comes to keeping your human machine out of trouble. Depending on whom you talk to, your body may be no more or less complex and difficult to handle and maintain than a complicated aircraft. To trust only a physician's statement that you are healthy enough to fly an airplane, rather than relying on a complete appraisal of airworthiness, is not realistic. As I stated before, some physicians are not overly familiar with the medical standards necessary to be a safe pilot, the reasons for them, or the effect on a pilot's performance if they are not met. Therefore, the medical criteria that must be met by each pilot are documented in writing in FAR Part 67 and then further defined for the AME in the *Guide for Aviation Medical Examiners*—both revised in 1996. Just as your aircraft specs need to be checked, your physiological and psychological specs must be documented so that you and others can be assured that you're fit to fly.

The medical specs have one characteristic in your favor: the majority of the medical criteria are guidelines for doctors and the FAA to follow. There is no hard and fast rule regarding the individual pilot. This allows aeromedical physicians and the FAA some flexibility, because they can review each case on its own merits. They then pass judgment, medically speaking, only on the individual patient's ability to be a safe pilot while flying. You need not be in perfect health—just medically safe. For example, there are acceptable limits for blood pressure in medical publications and the old FAR Part 67. No pilot is judged by a doctor or the FAA as having "hypertension" until that pilot is fully evaluated and several blood pressure readings have been taken. However, if an AME doesn't provide the FAA with these data and submits just one high blood pressure reading (even though it is only slightly above the expected maximums), there can be only one initial conclusion by the FAA—the pilot has high blood pressure (or hypertension) until proven otherwise.

The FAA has one medical goal in defining the medical standards that all pilots must meet: to ensure that each pilot is free of any medical problem that would interfere with the safe performance of duties while flying. The U.S. military differs in its regulations in that it spells out potential medical deficiencies far more elaborately than does the FAA. This is appropriate for the military flight surgeon system since the flight surgeon has more direct authority than the AME and there must be no doubt that each military pilot throughout the world is being adequately evaluated and meets strict, well-defined standard criteria. It used to be that the military medically certified its pilots for all its aircraft—all or none. The FAA, on the other hand, could functionally limit the operations of an aircraft on the medical certificate and thus allow some pilots to fly with a medical problem but only in certain crew positions. However, years ago this was reversed. The military now medically qualifies pilots for specific aircraft whereas the FAA has been instructed by the courts that it cannot limit functional operations for first-class medicals. The rule, however, allows for functional limitations for second- and third-class medicals.

THE PILOT AS FLIGHT SURGEON

The keys to the FAA's medical certification policy are FAR 61.53

OPERATIONS DURING MEDICAL DEFICIENCY:
NO PERSON MAY ACT AS PILOT IN COMMAND, OR IN ANY OTHER CAPACITY AS A REQUIRED PILOT FLIGHT CREW MEMBER WHILE HE HAS A KNOWN MEDICAL DEFICIENCY, OR INCREASE OF A KNOWN MEDICAL DEFICIENCY THAT WOULD MAKE HIM UNABLE TO MEET THE REQUIREMENTS FOR HIS CURRENT MEDICAL CERTIFICATE.

and FAR 91.11(a)(3)

NO PERSON MAY ACT AS A CREW MEMBER OF A CIVIL AIR-
CRAFT WHILE USING ANY DRUG THAT AFFECTS HIS FACULTIES
IN ANY WAY CONTRARY TO SAFETY.

FAR Part 61, by the way, seems to be in a continuous state of revision because it is so broad in its coverage. FAR 61.53 is one regulation that won't be
rewritten but may be supplemented by other limitations that the pilot must follow. The intent is the same.

Basically, these regulations mean that the decision to fly as a safe pilot is
on your shoulders. They are based on the assumption that you will accept the
responsibility of being in good health and ground yourself should you develop
a medical impairment (*deficiency*). The problem, of course, is knowing if you
have a medical deficiency and if it affects your flying. Your medical education
in flight training, ground school, and recurrent training is minimal at best. How
are you expected to know if that pain in your chest is significant or why you
can't fly with high blood pressure?

Keep in mind that you have the right to fly at any time while you carry a
valid medical certificate, provided you can comply with FAR 61.53 and FAR
91.11(a)(3). In fact, look on the back of your medical certificate. You'll see a
clear reminder to consider FAR 61.53 as your responsibility while you are a
crew member! Also keep in mind that this is Part 61, which applies to pilots, as
opposed to Part 67, the medical criteria used by doctors. You could look at this
as meaning that Part 67 is used to assist in the interpretation of the requirements that must be met in 61.53.

There is nothing mysterious about the content of Part 67 of the FARs.
However, I have seen a variety of interpretations by attorneys, physicians, pilots, and other "authorities." Many of these interpretations are misleading or
incomplete—and most leave you with more questions unanswered than answered, assuming you knew what questions to ask in the first place! And the revised and amended 1996 standards add fuel to that discussion with new
material to challenge. Once again, let me state that there is a medical reason
for every one of these medical regulations or standards but they are intended
for use by doctors, not pilots, although they obviously have a direct effect on
you. The *legal* interpretation is a matter for the courts and the National Transportation Safety Board (NTSB).

When going through Part 67, it is important for you to realize that, except
for several well-defined, specific medical disorders to be explained later, the
regulations are vague—for a reason: this allows the FAA to judge your medical
problem on an individual basis and to interpret all available medical data, thus

allowing reconsiderations, waivers, Statements of Demonstrated Ability (SODAs), and limitations, even though your health may not meet the letter of the law. Compare this with Part 121, which is rarely waived (the age sixty retirement rule is under Part 121 and therefore cannot be waived).

Part 67 basically defines medical standards that must be met for first-, second-, and third-class medical certificates. The protocol is the same for each level, but the range of acceptable limits differs in a few situations. In other words, the exam should be the same for every pilot for any class—the limits you must meet depend on the class for which you are applying. The medical criteria as they pertain to a first-class certificate are listed in the paragraph 67.100 series (the old 67.13), which I discuss in this book; the second- and third-class requirements are less stringent variations of the same basic criteria.

(Part of the 1996 amendments to Part 67 include a complete revision of the coding numbers. This is further explained in Appendix I. For clarification, both codings are stated in this text, with the old code in parentheses.)

MANDATORY (INITIAL) DENIALS

Before we go into the regulations that govern the more common but less serious medical deficiencies, let's discuss the medical conditions for which certification denial is mandatory by the Aviation Medical Examiner. They are listed separately here since they pose the greatest threat to a pilot's career. The remainder of FAR Part 67 is listed in Appendix I, with an explanation of each item. I encourage you to scan the appendix to be familiar with its contents.

Note that at the end of a major section in FAR Part 67 (e.g., the mental, neurological, or general medical condition section) there is a generic statement defining that

> a pilot can have no other [disorder as is being defined]. ... that the Federal Air Surgeon, based on the case history and appropriate, qualified medical judgment relating to the condition involved, finds the person unable to safely perform the duties or exercise the privileges of the airman certificate [note: not the medical certificate but the flying certificate] applied for or held or may reasonably be expected, for the maximum duration of the airman medical certificate applied for or held, to make the person unable to perform those duties or exercise those privileges.

This is a blanket standard that covers any other disorder that is not specifically stated in FAR Part 67 that could be an unacceptable risk in flight. Some pilots think this gives the FAA too much control, but in reality, there is no way that all disorders can be listed. Remember, FAR Part 67 gives the FAA the authority to determine what is safe and unsafe without being an unmanageable textbook of medical problems. The bottom line is that the FAA will certify you if you can prove you are an acceptable risk in flight.

The majority of the medical disorders described relate to the current status of the disorder. That is, if you have a broken leg, you can't fly while it is healing, but once it has healed, there is no problem with flying. It's a different story for the disorders that require a mandatory denial. It is important to note that these regulations state that even an established medical *history* of any of the conditions means a mandatory initial denial by the AME. For example, if you had a heart problem twenty years ago that has since been completely resolved, a mandatory denial would still be required. As we will see, this mandatory denial by the AME sets the stage for further evaluation and collection of data to allow the FAA (not the AME) to judge whether or not you can fly safely. Most of the reasoning behind denying certification to a pilot with a history of any one of these disorders should be self-explanatory, but the relationship of the severity of the disorder to its effect on your flying ability is often misunderstood or underrespected. Therefore, I will take each one individually and attempt to clarify the justification for the initial denial. At one time there were nine disorders that led to an automatic denial. This list has been expanded to the "fearful fifteen." The additional disorders have always been cause for denial but were buried in the regulations. The following interpretations are my own and do not necessarily represent those of the FAA.

Conditions for Which Certificate Denial Is Mandatory

Each of these disorders is clearly defined as a distinct FAR, which usually begins with "No established medical history or clinical diagnosis of" in subparagraph a.

1. FAR 67.107(a)(1) A PERSONALITY DISORDER WHICH IS SEVERE ENOUGH TO HAVE REPEATEDLY MANIFESTED ITSELF BY OVERT ACTS (old FAR 67.13[d][1][i][a])

We all know people who, in our own judgment, do strange things at strange times. This does not necessarily mean that they are mentally ill or that they have a severe mental disease requiring medication and psychiatric therapy. If a pilot has a personality disorder that could interfere with his or her performance as a crew member and the pilot cannot exercise self-control in situations requiring his or her full attention, the pilot's outbursts would be considered "overt acts" that could reappear at inopportune times. Obviously this is a tough regulation to define, quantify, and apply to an individual pilot, and it is difficult to evaluate and document. It calls for subjective judgment and clear proof that the disorder would compromise safe flying. For example, the pilot being afraid to fly in bad weather or outwardly antagonistic toward company policies is not in itself unsafe, but in bad weather or when morale must be maintained on the flight deck, the results could be disastrous. At what point is the pilot's behavior hazardous? Who should establish that point?

2. FAR 67.107(a)(2) A PSYCHOSIS (old FAR 67.13[d][1][i][b])

In the eyes of the FAA, this means the individual has "manifested delusions, hallucinations, grossly bizarre or disorganized behavior, or other commonly accepted symptoms of this condition," or the individual may reasonably be expected to manifest the same symptoms.

Medically speaking, someone who is psychotic is definitely mentally ill. There are many types of psychotic disorders, with names you've heard like "split personality," "paranoid," or "schizophrenic." These disorders are characterized by withdrawal from reality and an inability to cope with the usual stresses of life, certainly not the pressures of a pilot. Psychoses usually require treatment, which may include hospitalization, medication, and continuous psychiatric therapy. It is not difficult for a psychiatrist to diagnose and document a pilot who is clearly psychotic. However, there is much skepticism in the pilot community concerning psychiatry and psychology. I doubt, however, that any responsible pilot would allow a clearly psychotic pilot to fly either as a crew member or alone.

3. FAR 67.107(a)(3) A BIPOLAR DISORDER (new standard)

Although new, this disorder (equivalent to manic-depressive) has always been included under mental problems, but because of its change in the medical "code" books, it is now added as a specifically disqualifying condition.

4. FAR 67.107(a)(4) SUBSTANCE DEPENDENCE (old ALCOHOLISM [FAR 67.13(d)(1)(i)(c)])

This used to be called alcoholism, but over the years there has been an increased awareness of and testing for other chemicals of dependency. This will be explained more fully in the chapter on certification. For now, the definition of *substance* includes alcohol, sedatives, hypnotics (sleeping medication), antidepressants, and other legal and illicit drugs and inhalants. Dependence, as will be described later, means a condition in which a person is dependent on a substance as evidenced by increased tolerance, withdrawal symptoms, and impaired control of use.

This subject has been drawing a lot of attention in recent years, especially with the new testing requirements and new treatment and recertification of dependence. This has resulted in marked changes in the FAA's consideration for recertifying rehabilitated alcoholics. It used to be that someone with a history of being an alcoholic, even if it was twenty-five years ago, could never fly again. This has changed thanks to the combined efforts of ALPA (Airline Pilot's Association) and the FAA. After adequate therapy, "tincture of time," and documentation of sobriety along with an ongoing surveillance program, the FAA will consider certifying a former abuser of alcohol. The problem, of course, is in identifying and diagnosing a pilot as truly being a chronic drinker. The medical and mental professions are learning more about how to define a pilot who actually is an alcoholic and how to determine whether or not he or she is a heavy social drinker or frequent abuser of alcohol. Alcoholism is chronic. It is a disease. The recent amendment now states medical certification is denied "except where there is established clinical evidence, satisfactory to the Federal Air Surgeon, of recovery, including sustained total abstinence from the substance(s) for not less than the preceding 2 years." This allows for certification after proper documentation. The two-year period can also be reconsidered through FAR 67.401 (the old 67.19) "special issuance of medical certificate" so that a recovering alcoholic can be returned to flying much sooner.

The old 67.13 covering drug dependence (FAR 67.13[d][1][i][d]) is now included in the preceding new rule (67.107[a][4]). This inclusion is straightforward since, if you will recall, FAR 91.11 states pilots should use no drugs of any kind that could affect their ability to fly. Although this usually implies narcotics, this also could mean any drug, even nonprescription, over-the-counter medications. Even though we may be able to tolerate a specific drug on the ground, the effects of that drug can change dramatically at altitude and under stress. Here again, I do not think too many responsible pilots would want a crew member who could not function without drugs.

The amended standards describe the criteria the FAA uses to initiate any questioning of a pilot's potential dependence. Furthermore, in addressing the issue of its expectations for recertifying the substance-dependent pilot, the FAA states in the discussion section of Part 67:

> In many cases, the FAA has granted special issuance to air transport and commercial pilots and has waived the 2-year abstinence period when it was satisfied that certain stringent criteria are met. The criteria can be summarized as follows: (1) a full commitment and partnership of the aviation employer and employee to ensure

the employee's continued sobriety through monitoring; (2) full commitment and partnership of the recovering employee with a fellow employee to ensure continued sobriety through monitoring; and (3) frequent evaluations, testing, and attendance at professional aftercare treatment.

Additionally, the FAR (as noted in the statement before this part) states that a pilot can have no other personality disorder, neurosis, or mental condition that the Federal Air Surgeon judges will interfere with the pilot's ability to fly safely.

5. FAR 67.107(b) SUBSTANCE ABUSE (new)

This new addition to the mandatory denials is further elaborated in the FAR: there should be no substance abuse within the preceding two years, no verified positive drug test result, no misuse of a substance that makes the person unable to perform the duties of a pilot, and no defined use of a substance in a situation in which that use was physically hazardous, for example, as evidenced by a DUI (driving under the influence) or DWI (driving while intoxicated). The *Guide for Aviation Medical Examiners* suggests that this FAR is enforced if there has been substance abuse within two years of a previous abuse. In other words, the first DUI or DWI is usually disregarded, but a second occurrence is not.

6. FAR 67.109(a)(1) EPILEPSY (old FAR 67.13[d][2][i][a])

The dilemma with this standard is based on the *history* of epilepsy (a convulsion or seizure disorder that can recur at any unexpected time). For example, if you had a convulsion even as a child, such as a "fever convulsion," this is technically disqualifying until proven completely resolved. What is difficult to determine is whether or not the individual will have another epileptic seizure. Medically speaking, a person who has had a convulsive attack of any kind has a greater chance of having another one at any time. Obviously, if medication is required to control the epilepsy, this use of the drug is also disqualifying.

7. FAR 67.109(a)(2) DISTURBANCE OF CONSCIOUSNESS WITHOUT SATISFACTORY MEDICAL EXPLANATION OF THE CAUSE (old FAR 67.13[d][2][i][b])

This includes that mild concussion you had back in high school as a football player. Pilots who have the potential for losing consciousness are obviously not qualified to be crew members. A physician cannot guarantee, unless all tests indicate otherwise, that an individual who has had any kind of disturbance of consciousness in the past will not have another occurrence. Unfortunately, medical science does not always come up with a specific answer to why a pilot has a disturbance of consciousness. Doctors can say what you don't have but may not be able to say what you do have. Therefore, you are left with a problem with no known cause or explanation! To almost anyone other than a pilot, this would not be a problem. In your case, passage of time, often years, is necessary before a doctor can reconsider the chances of a recurrence. However, if, as in a history of a mild concussion, the neurological evaluation is normal and there is a satisfactory explanation that proves the concussion's insignificance, the FAA will usually consider the application favorably.

8. FAR 67.109(a)(3) TRANSIENT LOSS OF CONTROL OF NERVOUS SYSTEM FUNCTION(S) WITHOUT SATISFACTORY MEDICAL EXPLANATION OF THE CAUSE (new rule)

This is an extension of the loss of consciousness standards but includes other neurological disorders beyond loss of consciousness, such as significant numbness, tremors, and other disorders that are an obvious impairment when happening. The key point is that something like this is unexplained. If there is no cause, it can't be fixed, removed, or (probably) controlled.

9. FAR 67.111(a)(1) MYOCARDIAL INFARCTION (old FAR 67.13[e][1][i])

This is straightforward but often misunderstood. Why can't a pilot fly simply because he or she had a heart attack (myocardial infarction) five years ago—especially when this person is in better shape and better health now than ever before? The reason is that, statistically speaking, that pilot still has a greater chance of having a heart attack than a pilot who has not had one, especially at altitude, even if the medical risk factors (such as hypertension, smoking, and elevated cholesterol) have been eliminated. (This will be discussed later.) The FAA, however, is reconsidering the applications of pilots with heart attack histories, even for first class, after passage of at least six months. In some cases patients have been misdiagnosed as having had a heart attack when, in fact, they had some other medical problem, such as pericarditis or a variation on an ECG or other test. Therefore, if pilots have had a heart attack, this is disqualifying until it can be proven they have had no residual disease, they have no current problems with their hearts or coronary arteries, and they have no cardiac risk factors that would allow the disease to progress.

As a part of the medical evaluation for a first-class medical certificate the FAA requires an ECG at certain ages. It is first required at age thirty-five, then at age forty, and then annually. One of the reasons for this is to show the absence of a previous undetected heart attack. By the way, the 1996 amendments do not require an ECG for second class, contrary to expectations.

10. FAR 67.111(a)(2) ANGINA PECTORIS (old FAR 67.13[e][1][ii])

11. FAR 67.111(a)(3) CORONARY HEART DISEASE THAT HAS REQUIRED TREATMENT OR, IF UNTREATED, THAT HAS BEEN SYMPTOMATIC OR CLINICALLY SIGNIFICANT (old FAR 67.13[e][1][ii])

This regulation covers a multitude of potential problems. The key here is the evidence of disease in one or more of the coronary arteries (arteries that carry blood to the heart muscle itself). The only way this can be disproved is with an angiogram (an X ray of the coronary arteries), which is not usually recommended by a doctor as a routine test. There are now evaluations, such as the thallium scan, echocardiogram, and CAT scan, that are less of a risk but still expensive. And, though they are becoming more accurate, they are not conclusive. The presence of coronary artery disease is serious and is sometimes manifested by severe and disabling chest pain called *angina,* which occurs when the heart muscle is not receiving an adequate supply of oxygen necessary to function properly. By the way, not all heart disease has pain. There are "silent" heart attacks. Therefore, in a physically demanding situation, when the heart is required to work even harder, it may fail, especially in hypoxic conditions. When ischemia (reduced blood supply to the heart muscle) is found on any ECG tracing, the FAA will probably not certify the pilot because of the unpredictability of ischemia's progression.

A dilemma develops, for example, when a pilot has high blood pressure for any number of reasons and the FAA therefore requires a complete cardiovascular evaluation. As a part of this evaluation, an exercise cardiac stress ECG (stress test) may be necessary. This test could indicate the pilot may have coronary artery disease or ischemia. Now the pilot faces two possible disqualifying conditions: high blood pressure and the stress-test abnormality—which could be a normal variation. This topic will be more fully discussed later; suffice it to say for now that coronary artery disease is a bona fide risk factor if actually present.

12. FAR 67.111(a)(4) CARDIAC VALVE REPLACEMENT

13. FAR 67.111(a)(5) PERMANENT CARDIAC PACEMAKER IMPLANTATION

14. FAR 67.111(a)(6) HEART REPLACEMENT

These three cardiac conditions are new specific regulations and are specified as mandatory denials. They have always been cause for disqualification in the generic "blanket" statement, but the FAA has chosen to specify these situations so as not to minimize their importance. These conditions do increase the risk of problems in flight.

15. 67.113(a) DIABETES MELLITUS THAT REQUIRES INSULIN OR OTHER HY-POGLYCEMIC DRUG FOR CONTROL (old FAR 67.13[f][1])

Diabetes is a disease that is poorly understood even by the medical profession. (This is another topic that will be discussed later and in Appendix III.) The FAA assumes that the pilot's physician who makes the diagnosis of diabetes and prescribes drugs for it is sure of that diagnosis, has tried all other means to control it, and is left with insulin or oral hypoglycemics to control the diabetes. This is a sad situation for the inherently healthy pilot since the "new" diabetes more than likely is the mature onset type, which means it has developed in the later years because of poor diet and physical conditioning. The diabetes can't be ignored and requires therapy, but it is probably directly related to that pilot's poor habits. The burden is on the pilot to prove that it can be controlled through diet alone without insulin—which should have been done in the first place. Some oral hypoglycemic medications can be certified after control is obtained and complete documentation provided.

In November 1996, the FAA did issue a policy change for *third-class* medicals for diabetics on insulin. The special issuance criteria are quite complex, but there will be some pilots who can meet these standards. These expectations include proving no recurrent significant hypoglycemic reactions, the absence of diabetes-related medical complications, periodic blood sugar testing before and during flight, and a medical evaluation every three months. This new policy represents a major change in philosophy, and only time will tell if it is a realistic exception to the rule and an acceptable risk. Of special concern is the responsibility of CFIs who are training (or retraining) diabetic recreational pilots—what is their liability and how do they intervene if the student becomes dizzy or confused? If you are diabetic but feel you can meet these standards, ask for a more definitive explanation from an AME who is knowledgeable about these criteria.

A comment about the use of medication is in order. If a pilot requires medication to control a medical disorder, then it must be assumed that other measures have been tried and failed, such as diet and avoiding substance abuse. In other words, it's not the side effects of the medication alone that are disqualifying; it is the fact that you have a disorder severe enough to require the use of the medicine.

When an Aviation Medical Examiner detects any of the disorders just described, he or she is required to deny the pilot's application for certification and to submit the information to the FAA.

FAR 61.53 AND FLYING (OR NOT FLYING)

Keep this in mind: FAR 61.53 can also be interpreted to mean that if you have a medical deficiency you are not breaking any regulations if you do not fly, even if you don't report the problem. That is, if you ground yourself, nothing illegal is being done. However, trying to hide any disorder and continuing to fly is a serious breach of responsibility and *is* illegal. The FAA wants AMEs to report all medical problems to keep the few irresponsible sick pilots from flying.

A key point to remember is that if you are healthy nobody really cares, especially the FAA. Many of the criteria state that you must be free of a certain medical disorder, but they don't state that you have to be healthy. Because of the wording, it would appear that the AME and the FAA have a negative approach, as if they are only looking for something wrong (and consequently are "out to get you"). They are, but only in the sense of proving the absence of a medical problem that would interfere with your safe flying. If nothing can be found, then usually nothing is said.

We have considered the fifteen most important medical standards that must be met. The rest of Part 67 as it pertains to the first-class medical certificate and other classes can be found in Appendix I. Remember, the medical FARs are basically realistic and fair—if interpreted correctly by your doctor and your AME.

What we have discussed thus far are the specific regulations that deal with medical standards. Except for the designated medical problems requiring denial by the AME (yet still certifiable by the Federal Air Surgeon), the rest of these FARs are not specific; that is, they are expressed in general terms. Therefore the AME uses a manual entitled *Guide for Aviation Medical Examiners,* published by the FAA to assist the doctor in complying with the FARs. This publication lists some of the specific medical disorders that would deny or defer certification. This guide also addresses specific parameters, such as blood pressure readings, for certain medical disorders, and parameters not identified in the FARs.

Once again, keep in mind that although the healthy pilot gets little recognition, the healthy pilot or the one who is an acceptable risk in flight is the only pilot an AME can certify. In essence, the medical examiner is evaluating the applicant to prove the absence of any medical disorder that would create a hazard to flying. The AME can defer the issuance of the certificate, which means that although an applicant may have a medical problem that person is not necessarily permanently grounded although he or she can't fly now. Once the applicant has been deferred or reported to the FAA, additional information from tests not normally a part of the usual FAA exam must be completed and reviewed by the FAA before the applicant can be certified. The medical examiner, therefore, has only the responsibility of proving during his or her examination that the applicant does not have any of the medical disqualifications noted in the guide. If the applicant has a potentially disqualifying medical problem, only the FAA can certify him or her. Current FAA policy does give the AME more authority if certain tests are normal.

Appendix II has a complete listing of the different specific items that must be evaluated and commented on by the medical examiner. The list follows the same order as on FAA Form 8500-8 (your application for medical certification). The list does not include all the possible medical disorders that would interfere with flying safely nor is it cast in concrete. That is, many of the listed conditions can be certified after an adequate evaluation and review by the FAA.

Read Appendix II if a specific disorder or medical condition interests you. For now, it is important to remember that this partial list is what you are judged by. You must be able to meet the standards every time you fly. Since you can't take a physical every day, you must play doctor and decide if you are safe to fly (we are back to FAR 61.53, which states you can't fly if you know you have a medical disorder).

Another important point is that the burden really is on you to further elaborate on a medical disorder. In other words, the FAA corresponds with you, not the AME. The reason is that you have the choice of seeing whichever doctor you want. The examiner can coordinate the evaluation and make the whole process more efficient for you, but reporting to the FAA or AME is still your responsibility.

One final item in Form 8500-8 is that section filled out by the examiner (item 61 in the old form; item 60 in the new 1992 form)—comments on history and findings. This is an area where Aviation Medical Examiners could forego many delays in the certification process; if they would just take the time to explain an abnormality found in the evaluation or supplement the data with other tests or reports from specialists, a lot of time and confusion could be saved. However, it is much easier for some examiners to simply submit brief medical data to the FAA and then let the FAA be the one to ask you for more data, come up with the conclusion, and be the "bad guy." This could be avoided in many cases if the examiner provided an explanation and the expected additional information to the FAA.

The medical history checked off by the pilot applicant on the front of FAA Form 8500-8 and the examination report by the AME on the back constitute the information sent to the FAA. If everything fits into the proper criteria and all the blanks are filled in, the local examiner can certify. However, he or she has no authority to certify if the applicant does not meet these criteria unless further evidence is provided to and approved by the FAA. The AME's guide helps you and the AME with these tests.

Keep in mind that the standards, criteria, and guidelines are used to determine if you are qualified to fly from day to day just as if you were asked to pass your physical every day prior to a trip. The key, once again, is FAR 61.53. If you are healthy—OK—go flying. If you're not healthy, then what? Any medical impairment is subject to interpretation by your doctor, your AME, and the FAA. If there is no potential problem in regard to your flying responsibility, there is no reason why you cannot be certified.

Every condition of Part 67 is subject to interpretation, and the Federal Air

Surgeon has the authority and flexibility to make judgment decisions. If you are considered safe to fly based on your current examination, the Federal Air Surgeon's office can certify you. This is why it is vitally important that those who sit in judgment be provided with as much pertinent information as possible to enable them to reach a responsible conclusion. Inadequate or incomplete reports will be looked upon as simply that. The FAA will return a judgment stating, "based on the information received," and it will state its conclusion, often not one that the pilot wants.

THE PILOT'S ROLE IN CERTIFICATION

We've all heard "war stories" from friends and peers that would contradict my original comment that the medical criteria of the FAA are fair. However, if the full truth were known about the circumstances in each case, one actually would find that inadequate information was supplied or that the applicant was not really aware of the significance of the disorder and did not understand its implications for safe flying. These war stories are not valid scientific data. More than likely, that grounded pilot judged OK by other pilots or even some doctors should, in reality, not be flying.

My sole purpose for reminding you of this is not to justify the FAA's actions but rather to encourage you to disregard what you hear in the rumor mill and to pursue evaluation of a medical disorder, either known or suspected, with competent aeromedical physicians who are aware of FAA protocol and requirements. They should personally assist you in acquiring the necessary documentation to justify your certification before making reports to the FAA.

You will note that the FARs and the *Guide for Aviation Medical Examiners* specify that the applicant is the one who is responsible for resolving a medical disorder. The point is that you, the pilot, must know where you truly stand medically and what your options are in terms of your required evaluation. It is up to you to ensure that any disorder that has been found is expeditiously and efficiently handled.

IN REVIEW

1. All disqualifying disorders can interfere with safe flying.

2. The added risk of a possible recurrence of those disorders often complicates the FAA's final judgment.

3. Simply because there are no symptoms doesn't mean you are not a potential risk or don't have a problem. It is up to the AME and the FAA to ensure that no problem exists.

4. In the absence of a disorder that would be hazardous to flying, and with adequate valid data, you can fly. You need not be in perfect health.

5. If you suspect you have a problem or you bust a physical, no report need be made to the FAA—if you don't fly.

6. When you can prove your good health, then the report is submitted to the FAA, and if you are an acceptable risk, you should be certified.

7. The FAA corresponds with you, the pilot—not the AME—for any additional workup. Therefore, you are responsible for maintaining your flying status.

8. A denial is not final unless you accept it as final. You can always be reconsidered.

3

The FAA's Certification Process

A forty-year-old corporate pilot had seen the same AME
for years without any mention of problems. However,
this time his AME was not available and he saw another
AME who was more thorough and detected a heart murmur. This doctor stated that the murmur was not significant, but the doctor also stated that she wasn't familiar
with what the FAA wanted; consequently, she did not
certify the pilot and submitted the data to the FAA. The
pilot was grounded, didn't know where to go, and had
to wait four weeks to hear from the FAA. Eventually,
after three months of seeing specialists and sending in
reports, he was flying again. The murmur couldn't be ignored, but the pilot need not have been grounded for
four months.

Flying is almost a sixth sense to you. You're a good "stick
and rudder" pilot. In fact, you rarely have to think about
what you are doing with your hands and feet as you "drive" your machine
down the ILS. Remember way back when you began flying? It took a long time
and a lot of practice and experience before you got this basic straight-and-level
act together, and your steep turns were anything but coordinated. While you
are recalling those exciting days, consider this: How would you explain to me
in writing the procedure for executing a coordinated standard-rate turn? It's
very difficult since you can't expect me to understand what you are describing
without my already knowing the basics of flying, let alone how the plane feels.
The only way to be sure that I can comprehend what you are describing is to
have me read your description more than once and then experience the turn.

I want you to be as familiar with how you are medically certified as you
are with the basic techniques of flying. Consequently, I face a similar problem
in describing the certification process. Next to the chapters on your own health
maintenance program, this chapter is probably the most important guide to
keeping your certification. But I can't expect you to comprehend what I am describing without assuming that you already know about part of this certification
process. To be sure that I keep this subject clear, I will add personal comments

based on years of experience to the description of the actual protocol of the process.

We established that a monitoring program is necessary to ensure that only healthy and/or safe pilots control aircraft. The FAA has this responsibility and as a result has developed a list of medical conditions potentially incompatible with safe flying. These conditions are discussed in other chapters. This chapter describes (1) how you are medically evaluated to determine the presence or absence of these conditions and (2) the administrative sequence of the certification process, including reconsiderations and appeals if you fail the physical. This generic process must be followed no matter what the medical condition is. Specific problems are described in FARs Part 67 and the *Guide for Aviation Medical Examiners* (see Appendixes I and II).

THE CERTIFICATION PROCESS IN GENERAL

The Medical Application and Examination

You must go to a designated FAA Aviation Medical Examiner—the AME of your choice—for the FAA physical. This AME is a physician designated by the FAA to provide the medical data with which the FAA can pass judgment. When you arrive for each FAA exam, you are, in effect, applying anew, as if this was the first time. The FAA Form 8500-8 (Application for Airman Medical Certificate) is the first step in applying to the FAA for a medical certificate. This form was updated in 1992 but was not changed when FAR Part 67, "Medical Standards and Certification," was revised in 1996.

Obviously, information on past applications is considered by the FAA, but at the time you are in the AME's office, you are essentially reapplying. You are asking the FAA to certify you as being healthy—or at least an acceptable risk—based on this medical information and the authority of your AME. If you do not meet the FAA criteria, the AME cannot certify you unless the FAA has granted its approval or given the authority to the AME.

Therefore, if there are no disqualifying conditions noted during your medical examination, you are promptly certified for the period of your medical classification. First class is for six months, second is for twelve months, and third is for thirty-six months until age forty, then it's good for twenty-four months. Most pilots do not think much about their medical status in the interim and do little to prepare themselves for the next FAA exam until just before they show up at the AME's office.

Keep in mind that although you have a current medical certificate in your pocket, you remain subject to FAR 61.53—you can't fly with a known medical problem. Regardless of when you passed your last physical, if you know that you are not healthy enough to fly, then you can't fly until your health and

Copy of FAA Form 8500-9 (Medical Certificate) or FAA Form 8420-2 Medical/Student Pilot Certificate) issued.

EE- 1195951

MEDICAL CERTIFICATE _____ **CLASS**
AND STUDENT PILOT CERTIFICATE

This certifies that (*Full name and address*):

void

Date of Birth	Ht.	Wt.	Hair	Eyes	Sex

has met the medical standards prescribed in Part 67, Federal Aviation Regulations, for this class of Medical Certificate.

Limitations

Date of Examination	Examiner's Serial No

Signature

Typed Name

AIRMAN'S SIGNATURE

---

1. Application For:
☐ Airman Medical Certificate   ☐ Airman Medical and Student Pilot Certificate

2. Class of Medical Certificate Applied For:
☐ 1st   ☐ 2nd   ☐ 3rd

3. Last Name _____ **First Name** _____ **Middle Name**

4. Social Security Number ___ - ___ - ___

5. Address _____ **Telephone Number**
Number/Street _____ ( )
City _____ State/Country _____ Zip Code

6. Date of Birth M M D D Y Y

7. Color of Hair   **8. Color of Eyes**   **9. Sex**

10. Type of Airman Certificate(s) Held:
☐ None   ☐ ATC Specialist   ☐ Flight Instructor   ☐ Recreational
☐ Airline Transport   ☐ Flight Engineer   ☐ Private   ☐ Other
☐ Commercial   ☐ Flight Navigator   ☐ Student

11. Occupation _____ **12. Employer**

13. Has Your FAA Airman Medical Certificate Ever Been Denied, Suspended, or Revoked?
☐ Yes   ☐ No   If yes, give date ___ ___   M M   Y Y

Total Pilot Time (Civilian only)   **16. Date of Last FAA Medical Application**
14. To Date   **15. Past 6 months**   ☐ No Prior Application   M M Y Y

17. Do You Currently Use Any Medication (Prescription or Nonprescription)?
☐ Yes   If yes, give name, purpose, dosage, and frequency.
☐ No

---

18. Medical History — Have you ever had or have you now any of the following? Answer "yes" for every condition you have ever had in your life. In the EXPLANATION box below, you may note "PREVIOUSLY REPORTED, NO CHANGE" only if the explanation of the condition was reported on a prior application for an airman medical certificate and there has been no change in your condition. **See Instructions Page**

Yes	No	Condition	Yes	No	Condition	Yes	No	Condition
a. ☐	☐	Frequent or severe headaches	g. ☐	☐	Heart or vascular trouble	m. ☐	☐	Mental disorders of any sort; depression, anxiety, etc.	r. ☐	☐	Military medical discharge
b. ☐	☐	Dizziness or fainting spell	h. ☐	☐	High or low blood pressure	n. ☐	☐	Substance dependence or failed a drug test ever; or substance abuse or use of illegal substance in the last 5 years.	s. ☐	☐	Medical rejection by military service
c. ☐	☐	Unconsciousness for any reason	i. ☐	☐	Stomach, liver, or intestinal trouble				t. ☐	☐	Rejection for life or health insurance
d. ☐	☐	Eye or vision trouble except glasses	j. ☐	☐	Kidney stone or blood in urine	o. ☐	☐	Alcohol dependence or abuse	u. ☐	☐	Admission to hospital
e. ☐	☐	Hay fever or allergy	k. ☐	☐	Diabetes	p. ☐	☐	Suicide attempt			See v. & w. Below
f. ☐	☐	Asthma or lung disease	l. ☐	☐	Neurological disorders; epilepsy, seizures, stroke, paralysis, etc.	q. ☐	☐	Motion sickness requiring medication	x. ☐	☐	Other illness, disability, or surgery

Conviction and/or Administrative Action History — See Instructions Page

Yes	No		Yes	No	
v. ☐	☐	History of (1) any conviction(s) involving driving while intoxicated by, while impaired by, or while under the influence of alcohol or a drug; or (2) history of any conviction(s) or administrative action(s) involving an offense(s) which resulted in the denial, suspension, cancellation, or revocation of driving privileges or which resulted in attendance at an educational or a rehabilitation program.	w. ☐	☐	History of nontraffic conviction(s) (misdemeanors or felonies).

Explanations: See Instructions Page

For FAA Use
Review Action Codes

---

19. Visits to Health Professional Within Last 3 Years. ☐ Yes (explain below) ☐ No   **See Instructions Page**

Date	Name, Address, and Type of Health Professional Consulted	Reason

---

- NOTICE -
Whoever in any matter within the jurisdiction of any department or agency of the United States knowingly and willfully falsifies, conceals or covers up by any trick, scheme, or device a material fact, or who makes any false, fictitious or fraudulent statements or representations, or entry, may be fined up to $250,000 or imprisoned not more than 5 years, or both. (18 U.S. Code Secs. 1001; 3571).

20. Applicant's National Driver Register and Certifying Declarations
I hereby authorize the National Driver Register (NDR), through a designated State Department of Motor Vehicles, to furnish to the FAA information pertaining to my driving record. This consent constitutes authorization for a single access to the information contained in the NDR to verify information provided in this application. Upon my request, the FAA shall make the information received from the NDR, if any, available for my review and written comment. Authority: 23 U.S. Code 401, Note.
NOTE: All persons using this form must sign it. NDR consent, however, does not apply unless this form is used as an application for Medical Certificate or Medical Certificate and Student Pilot Certificate.
I hereby certify that all statements and answers provided by me on this application form are complete and true to the best of my knowledge, and I agree that they are to be considered part of the basis for issuance of any FAA certificate to me. I have also read and understand the Privacy Act statement that accompanies this form.

Signature of Applicant _____ Date   M M D D Y Y

FAA Form 8500-8 (7-92) Supersedes Previous Edition.   **OMB Approval No. 2120-0034**

FAA Form 8500-8, Application for Airman Medical Certificate. The actual medical certificate is in the upper left-hand corner.

NOTE: FAA's Copy of the Report of Medical Examination Must be TYPED.

REPORT OF MEDICAL EXAMINATION

21. Height (inches)	22. Weight (pounds)	23. Statement of Demonstrated Ability (SODA)	24. SODA Serial Number
		☐ YES ☐ NO Defect Noted:	

CHECK EACH ITEM IN APPROPRIATE COLUMN	Normal	Abnormal	CHECK EACH ITEM IN APPROPRIATE COLUMN	Normal	Abnormal
25. Head, face, neck, and scalp			37. Vascular system (Pulse, amplitude and character; arms, legs, others)		
26. Nose			38. Abdomen and viscera (Including hernia)		
27. Sinuses			39. Anus (Not including digital examination)		
28. Mouth and throat			40. Skin		
29. Ears, general (Internal and external canals; Hearing under item 49)			41. G-U system (Not including pelvic examination)		
30. Ear Drums (Perforation)			42. Upper and lower extremities (Strength and range of motion)		
31. Eyes, general (Vision under items 50 to 54)			43. Spine, other musculoskeletal		
32. Ophthalmoscopic			44. Identifying body marks, scars, tattoos (Size & location)		
33. Pupils (Equality and reaction)			45. Lymphatics		
34. Ocular motility (Associated parallel movement, nystagmus)			46. Neurologic (Tendon reflexes, equilibrium, senses, cranial nerves, coordination, etc.)		
35. Lungs and chest (Not including breasts examination)			47. Psychiatric (Appearance, behavior, mood, communication, and memory)		
36. Heart (Precordial activity, rhythm, sounds, and murmurs)			48. General systemic		

NOTES: Describe every abnormality in detail. Enter applicable item number before each comment. Use additional sheets if necessary and attach to this form.

49. Hearing	Right Ear	Left Ear			Right Ear					Left Ear			
Voice Test			Audiometer Threshold in Decibels	500	1000	2000	3000	4000	500	1000	2000	3000	4000

50. Distant Vision	51. Near Vision	52. Color Vision
Right 20/ Corrected to 20/	Right 20/ Corrected to 20/	
Left 20/ Corrected to 20/	Left 20/ Corrected to 20/	
Both 20/ Corrected to 20/	Both 20/ Corrected to 20/	☐ Normal ☐ Abnormal

53. Field of Vision	54. Heterophoria 20' (in prism diopters)	Esophoria	Exophoria	Right Hyperphoria	Left Hyperphoria
☐ Normal ☐ Abnormal					

55. Blood Pressure	56. Pulse (Resting)	57. Urinalysis (if abnormal, give results)			58. ECG (Date)		
(Sitting, mm of Mercury) Systolic / Diastolic		☐ Normal ☐ Abnormal	Albumin	Sugar	MM	DD	YY

59. Other Tests Given

60. Comments on History and Findings: AME shall comment on all "YES" answers in the Medical History section and for abnormal findings of the examination. (Attach all consultation reports, ECGs, X-rays, etc. to this report before mailing.)

FOR FAA USE
Pathology Codes:

Coded By:

Clerical Reject

Significant Medical History ☐ YES ☐ NO   Abnormal Physical Findings ☐ YES ☐ NO

61. Applicant's Name	62. Has Been Issued — ☐ Medical Certificate ☐ Medical & Student Pilot Certificate
	☐ No Certificate Issued — Deferred for Further Evaluation
	☐ Has Been Denied — Letter of Denial Issued (Copy Attached)

63. Disqualifying Defects (List by item number)

64. Medical Examiner's Declaration — I hereby certify that I have personally reviewed the medical history and personally examined the applicant named on this medical examination report. This report with any attachment embodies my findings completely and correctly.

Date of Examination	Aviation Medical Examiner's Name	Aviation Medical Examiner's Signature
MM DD YY	Street Address	
		AME Serial Number
	City State Zip	AME Telephone ( )

FAA Form 8500-8 (7-92) Supersedes Previous Editions

32

Instructions for Completion of the Application for Airman Medical Certificate or Airman Medical and Student Pilot Certificate, FAA Form 8500-8

Applicant must fill in completely numbers 1 through 20 of the application using a ballpoint pen. Exert sufficient pressure to make legible copies. The following numbered instructions apply to the numbered headings on the application form that follows this page.

NOTICE — Intentional falsification may result in federal criminal prosecution. Intentional falsification may also result in suspension or revocation of all airman, ground instructor, and medical certificates and ratings held by you, as well as denial of this application for medical certification.

1. APPLICATION FOR — Check the appropriate box.

2. CLASS OF AIRMAN MEDICAL CERTIFICATE APPLIED FOR — Check the appropriate box for the class of airman medical certificate for which you are making application.

3. FULL NAME — If your name has changed for any reason, list current name on the application and list any former name(s) in the EXPLANATIONS box of number 18 on the application.

4. SOCIAL SECURITY NUMBER — The social security number is optional; however, its use as a unique identifier does eliminate mistakes.

5. ADDRESS — Give permanent mailing address and country. Include your complete nine digit ZIP code if known. Provide your current area code and telephone number.

6. DATE OF BIRTH — Specify month (MM), day (DD), and year (YY) in numerals; e.g., 01/31/50.

7. COLOR OF HAIR — Specify as brown, black, blond, gray, or red. If bald, so state. Do not abbreviate.

8. COLOR OF EYES — Specify actual eye color as brown, black, blue, hazel, gray, or green. Do not abbreviate.

9. SEX — Indicate male or female.

10. TYPE OF AIRMAN CERTIFICATE(S) HELD — Check applicable block(s). If "Other" is checked, provide name of certificate.

11. OCCUPATION — Indicate major employment. "Pilot" will be used only for those gaining their livelihood by flying.

12. EMPLOYER — Provide your employer's full name. If self-employed, so state.

13. HAS YOUR FAA AIRMAN MEDICAL CERTIFICATE EVER BEEN DENIED, SUSPENDED, OR REVOKED —If "yes" is checked, give month and year of action in numerals.

14. TOTAL PILOT TIME TO DATE — Give total number of civilian flight hours. Indicate whether logged or estimated. Abbreviate as Log. or Est.

15. TOTAL PILOT TIME PAST 6 MONTHS — Give number of civilian flight hours in the 6-month period immediately preceding date of this application. Indicate whether logged or estimated. Abbreviate as Log. or Est.

16. MONTH AND YEAR OF LAST FAA MEDICAL EXAMINATION —Give month and year in numerals. If none, so state.

17. DO YOU CURRENTLY USE ANY MEDICATION (Prescription or Nonprescription) — Check "yes" or "no." If "yes" is checked, give name of medication(s), purpose, dosage, and frequency (e.g., daily, twice daily, as needed, etc.). See **NOTE** below.

18. MEDICAL HISTORY — Each item under this heading must be checked either "yes" or "no." You must answer "yes" for every condition you have ever had in your life and describe the condition and approximate date in the EXPLANATIONS box.

If information has been reported on a previous application for airman medical certificate and there has been no change in your condition, you may note "PREVIOUSLY REPORTED, NO CHANGE" in the EXPLANATIONS box, but you must still check "yes" to the condition. Do not report occasional common illnesses such as colds or sore throats.

"Substance dependence" is defined by any of the following: increased tolerance; withdrawal symptoms; impaired control of use; or continued use despite damage to health or impairment of social, personal, or occupational functioning. "Substance abuse" includes the following: use of an illegal substance; use of a substance or substances in situations in which such use is physically hazardous; or misuse of a substance when such misuse has impaired health or social or occupational functioning. "Substances" include alcohol, PCP, marijuana, cocaine, amphetamines, barbiturates, opiates, and other psychoactive chemicals.

Conviction and/or Administrative Action History — Letter (v) of this subheading asks if you have ever been: (1) convicted (which may include paying a fine, or forfeiting bond or collateral) of an offense involving driving while intoxicated by, while impaired by, or while under the influence of alcohol or a drug; or (2) convicted or subject to an administrative action by a state or other jurisdiction for an offense for which your license was denied, suspended, cancelled, or revoked or for which you were required to attend an educational or rehabilitation program. Individual traffic convictions are not required to be reported if they did not involve: alcohol or a drug; suspension, revocation, cancellation, or denial of driving privileges; or attendance at an educational or rehabiltation program. If "yes" is checked, a description of the conviction(s) and/or administrative action(s) must be given in the EXPLANATIONS box. The description must include: (1) the alcohol or drug offense for which you were convicted or the type of administrative action involved (e.g., attendance at an alcohol treatment program in lieu of conviction; license denial, suspension, cancellation, or revocation for refusal to be tested; educational safe driving program for multiple speeding convictions; etc.); (2) the name of the state or other jurisdiction involved; and (3) the date of the conviction and/or administrative action. The FAA may check state motor vehicle driver licensing records to verify your responses. Letter (w) of this subheading asks if you have ever had any other (nontraffic) convictions (e.g., assault, battery, public intoxication, robbery, etc.). If so, name the charge for which you were convicted and the date of conviction in the EXPLANATIONS box. See **NOTE** below.

19. VISITS TO HEALTH PROFESSIONAL WITHIN LAST 3 YEARS— List all visits in the last 3 years to a physician, physician assistant, nurse practitioner, psychologist, clinical social worker, or substance abuse specialist for treatment, examination, or medical/mental evaluation. List visits for counseling only if related to a personal substance abuse or psychiatric condition. Give date, name, address, and type of health professional consulted and briefly state reason for consultation. Multiple visits to one health professional for the same condition may be aggregated on one line. Routine dental, eye, and FAA periodic medical examinations and consultations with your employer-sponsored employee assistance program (EAP) may be excluded unless the consultations were for your substance abuse or unless the consultations resulted in referral for psychiatric evaluation or treatment. See **NOTE** below.

20. APPLICANT'S DECLARATION — Two declarations are contained under this heading. The first authorizes the National Driver Register to release adverse driver history information, if any, about the applicant to the FAA. The second certifies the completeness and truthfulness of the applicant's responses on the medical application. The declaration section must be signed and dated by the applicant after the applicant has read it.

NOTE: If more space is required to respond to "yes" answers for numbers 17, 18, or 19, use a plain sheet of paper bearing the information, your signature, and the date signed.

Applicant—Please Tear Off This Sheet After Completing The Application Form.

FAA Form 8500-8 (7-92) Supersedes FAA Form 8500-12

fitness to fly is reviewed by the FAA or your AME. In other words, if you can't pass a flying physical on the day that you fly, then you can't legally or safely fly, even though you may have had a good physical evaluation two weeks before. Since you aren't a doctor or AME, it is often difficult for you to determine what needs to be done when you're not feeling right. (We'll discuss this predicament in detail later in this chapter.)

If at your examination something is not OK, a whole new process will begin, either to confirm your disqualification or to determine that the medical condition is not, in fact, a deterrent to safe flying. Suppose that a medical problem is detected, even though you haven't noticed any symptoms and you did not have the problem the last time you took the physical. The FAA will want more information. An important point to remember at this stage is that, unless your AME anticipates what the FAA needs and provides that information with Form 8500-8, the FAA will correspond with you, not the AME.

The FAA's Response to the Application

All applications, regardless of the results, are sent to the Aeromedical Certification Branch of the FAA in Oklahoma City. This office receives over 2,000 applications per day! Results of each application must be fed into the computer before any action is taken, a process that takes about two to three weeks. Any abnormal, incomplete, or equivocal application that suggests you aren't fit to fly has to be reviewed by a doctor, not the computer. The FAA doctor does not get the opportunity to pass judgment on an application until several weeks after it was mailed from an AME's office.

Furthermore, there are many applications on the doctor's desk that arrived before yours. It is no wonder there are delays in the certification process. Remember, you may know you have a problem and don't have a certificate with which to fly, but you must wait for the FAA's written response to your application before you can even begin to work toward getting your certificate back.

In the early 1990s, the FAA began using a computerized system for AMEs called the AeroMedical Certification Subsystem, or AMCS. This is a computer work station, located in the AME's office, on which the information from the application form is entered. The data are immediately compared with past data within the database, and the technician is alerted if there is a change. Furthermore, the computer program will prompt the technician if all the correct information has not been entered or if it isn't within acceptable standards. Explanations can be entered to satisfy the computer's requirements. Once everything is complete and accurate, the information is E-mailed to the FAA's aeromedical certification branch in Oklahoma City. If the AME has identified problems that could interfere with your ability to fly safely, you or the AME will need to submit additional information to the FAA's aeromedical doctors.

The AME's office should defer certification until these additional reports can be submitted. AMCS significantly speeds the medical certification process and ensures its completeness and accuracy. However, not all AMEs are using this system.

I would like to put in a few words for the physicians and their assistants in the Aeromedical Certification Branch of the FAA as well as the other aeromedical offices of the FAA. Contrary to what many pilots think, as indicated by the aviation press, these are caring people. They have no desire to ground you. A grounded pilot means more work for the FAA, something it doesn't need since it tends to be chronically behind in administrative duties. The FAA has an awesome responsibility to certify only those pilots who are not likely to become impaired while flying, now and in the immediate future.

Many pilots, with their careers hanging in the balance, feel that the bureaucracy of the FAA is and historically has been impersonal, uncaring, and downright unreasonable. This is not true of the medical personnel of the FAA. I know this because I have worked with these people and have seen them at work. They must follow bureaucratic rules and work within difficult limitations. If given the opportunity and the information to help the grounded pilot, the aeromedical certification people of the FAA will do their best to arrive at a fair yet responsible decision.

Many pilots will not agree with this observation and will have their own "war stories" to tell. However, if you knew all the facts about those cases, I doubt that you would find the FAA solely to blame for results considered unfair. The FAA doctors are not always right about a pilot, but they seldom are wrong in their decisions based on the data supplied to them!

Another misconception is that pilots' certificates may be taken away unnecessarily by the FAA while they are certified. Actually, this only happens when the FAA determines that pilots have a disqualifying condition after the AME has certified them and has already given them their medical certificates. The 1996-amended Part 67 states that the FAA must inform the pilot of the reversal within sixty days of its being issued by the AME. Usually, if a problem is noted in an AME exam, the certificate is simply not issued, and the pilot cannot legally fly. This is a picky point, but this misunderstanding contributes to the fear of the medical certification process.

The reason your certificate is pulled at a later date may not be the fault of the FAA. It may be that your AME failed to detect a problem later identified by the FAA when the medical data is reviewed by the FAA's doctors. The result, however, is the same: a grounded pilot. Your AME should tell you when you haven't passed the exam or when there is a potential problem instead of implying that everything is OK and forcing the FAA to "pull your ticket" later. If the evaluation is handled properly by the AME in the beginning, there is no need for the FAA to ground you after you've been certified.

If your AME denies your certification, you can appeal that decision within thirty days with the same information that was provided by the AME. However, it's important to keep in mind that, regardless of when you were issued the denial, if you acquire additional information or if enough time has passed for your disorder to improve the FAA will always reconsider your application at any time in the future.

Denied Examination/Application

After the FAA doctor in Oklahoma City has read your abnormal, incomplete, or equivocal application and finds that it is possibly disqualifying, he or she replies directly to you, either by requesting additional information or confirming the AME's denial. If you are denied, this letter fully explains the appeal procedures to you (there are several, as will be described).

If more information is required and an appeal is suggested, a time limit is stated, such as sixty days, depending on your medical condition and its effect on safe flying. The purpose of this is twofold: first, to identify how long your file will be kept active and your certificate kept valid by the FAA and, second, to determine how serious you are in pursuing your medical certification. There is a surprising number of denied pilots who don't follow up on what is required. In 1994, there were 2,916 denials (out of 452,992 applications), but of that number, 1,278 failed to pursue reconsideration, and another 1,116 failed to provide the FAA with the information needed to reach a conclusion. Therefore, only 522 pilots were denied based on a legitimate review of their cases (less than 0.12 percent of all applications!). The others still had a chance to prove their airworthiness.

Your file can be reopened at any time. For example, if a letter states that you have sixty days to respond, and you don't, the FAA interprets this to mean that you couldn't document that your medical condition was not disqualifying (and the FAA has no way of knowing this unless you send a report), that you haven't gotten all the information together yet, or that you are not interested in pursuing reconsideration of your medical certification.

After the deadline, you are no longer legally medically certified even if you have been certified by the AME. If you simply can't get the medical evaluation done before the deadline, you only have to submit the data to reopen your file and begin the appeal process again. Through your AME, you can call the FAA for an extension and explain why. If it is reasonable, the FAA might agree and allow you to keep flying during your evaluation.

In mid-1992, a new 8500-8 application form was released to replace all older forms. The intent was to revise areas that were not clear in the history section and to assist the medical examiner in his or her exam conclusions. (There were other changes that will be described later.) The main change in the new 8500-8 is the inclusion of an "express consent" declaration at the bottom of the application form. This provides authorization for the FAA to request traffic history information from the National Driver Register. If you do not sign and certify this part of the form, the medical certificate cannot be issued.

The reason behind this revision is the increasing awareness of pilots' illegal and unsafe use of alcohol and other drugs while flying. Of special concern is alcohol dependency, or alcoholism. The FAA recognizes that denial is a common symptom of dependency and that a pilot who is an alcoholic will not admit there is a problem to an AME or on an application. It is also recognized that an alcoholic's driving record often includes alcohol-related offenses. Several alcohol-related traffic tickets indicate that the driver (or pilot) is more than just a social drinker. Before the new Form 8500-8 came into effect, an interesting study showed that in Florida there were hundreds of pilots who still had their medical certificate to fly but couldn't drive to the airport because their driver's licenses had been revoked for driving under the influence. (More on this later.)

In item 18(v) of Form 8500-8, the FAA states it is looking for "History of (1) any conviction(s) involving driving while intoxicated by, while impaired by, or while under the influence of alcohol or a drug; or (2) history of any conviction(s) or administrative action(s) involving an offense(s) which resulted in the denial, suspension, cancellation, or revocation of driving privileges or which resulted in attendance at an educational or a rehabilitation program."

The FAA further explains, "Individual traffic convictions are not required to be reported if they did not involve: alcohol or a drug; suspension, revocation, cancellation, or denial of driving privileges; or attendance at an educational or rehabilitation program." If a conviction must be reported, a description of it or the administrative action must be given in the "Explanations" box.

In other words, the FAA wants to know about alcohol- or drug-related situations that could indicate that you have a substance abuse problem significant enough to affect your ability to fly safely.

Specifically, the applicant's declaration (see item 20) states: "I hereby authorize the National Driver Register (NDR), through a designated State Department of Motor Vehicles, to furnish to the FAA information pertaining to my driving record." Remember that Form 8500-8 is a legal document and how you respond on it is your responsibility. Your signature on the form confirms that what has been recorded is true.

Another area clarified on the new form is the definition of "seeing any health professional." The old form implied the health professional must be a physician. The new form states that the health professional may be a physician, physician assistant, nurse practitioner, psychologist, clinical social worker, or substance abuse specialist. Also, the period for reporting visits to the health professional has been reduced from five to three years. A visit includes treatment, examination, evaluation, or counseling. Initially, there was some confusion about what sort of counseling had to be reported. The FAA encourages the pilot to seek help for stress, marriage problems, and other situational problems. This sort of counseling *does not* need to be reported. However, if alcohol or drugs is a part of the problem or if medication is used as part of the treatment, then the counseling visits must be reported.

Even though you are probably familiar with the form, it is important to read the questions and the instructions that are attached. Be sure that every one of your affirmative answers is explained in section 17, section 19, or "Explanations," which follows 18(w). It is not necessary to spell out the explanation at each exam. Simply state, "Previously reported, no change" in the explanations box. You still must check the yes box; you just don't have to explain it every time. For item 19, once the three years are up and there have been no other visits to a health professional, then the no box can be checked.

The medical history section (item 18) is self-explanatory. Item 18(n), regarding substance use, is further explained by the FAA in the instruction sheet that accompanies the application form:

> "Substance dependence" is defined by any of the following: increased tolerance; withdrawal symptoms; impaired control of use; or continued use despite damage to health or impairment of social, personal, or occupational functioning. "Substance abuse" includes the following: use of an illegal substance; use of a substance or substances in situations in which such use is physically hazardous; or misuse of a substance when such misuse has impaired health or social or occupational functioning. "Substances" include alcohol, PCP, marijuana, cocaine, amphetamines, barbiturates, and other psychoactive chemicals.

Note that just using an illicit substance is reportable because it is illegal.

Testing for glaucoma (other than for field of vision), a digital rectal exam and female pelvic exam, and checking the exercise pulse are not necessary unless requested by the applicant. Another change in Form 8500-8 is that minor colds and illnesses need not be reported. In general, if there is any doubt about what to report, it is better to answer yes and then adequately explain that response in the explanations section. Don't assume the AME will clarify the situation; ask him or her to do it.

I suggest you review the form carefully, including the instructions (see page 33), before you sign it. In fact, take the instruction sheet home with you for future reference. You should review the AME's portion to ensure that the doctor understands his or her responsibilities. As will be described later, items 60 and 62 are critical since the AME has the chance to fully explain any findings that may be questioned by the FAA.

The Federal Air Surgeon in Washington, D.C., will pass judgment on more serious or complicated medical conditions that the Oklahoma City doctors or the Regional Flight Surgeons do not have authority to judge. However, the doctors in Oklahoma City now have more authority to certify special issuance files. These doctors will use the expertise of other specialists. It is important to recognize that many disqualifying conditions can be certified in Oklahoma City if you know what the FAA expects and submit the appropriate information. This is a critical point. The FAA doctors, wherever they are located, cannot act in your best interests unless provided with adequate medical reports. It would be like making a weather decision based only on the temperature and wind velocity. There is no way you can justify your decision of flying in adverse weather without more data. The FAA doctors have the same problem with your application if you and your AME have not "filled in all the squares" and provided the necessary additional tests and evaluations.

THE CERTIFICATION PROCESS IN DETAIL

Now that you have an overview of the process, let's go back to the beginning, to the point at which you walk into your AME's office. You can see any AME you choose, even a different one each time if you wish. Whether it is the first visit or the twentieth, the procedure used to certify you should be the same. However, the medical exam and the interpretation of its results can differ from one AME to another—and often does. For example, one AME may say you have an abnormal ECG. Another AME may claim that the ECG poses no problem. Only the FAA, in the final analysis, has the authority to decide, provided it is given enough of the right data. The more you know about how the process works *before* you sign the application, the more control you will have over the FAA's evaluation of it.

The Application and the AME

You first fill out the front part of FAA Form 8500-8. This part is self-explanatory and is similar to any other medical history section, such as in a standard insurance application. It could be tempting not to admit past or present conditions that you know or suspect will be disqualifying. I can't honestly disagree with the reasoning. Your career and right to fly are at stake, and you no doubt have thought, "Who's to know as long as I feel OK?" But deliberately hiding even a small abnormality on a legal form is unwise because you could be, in fact, threatening your career if you have a potentially dangerous medical condition, and you would be falsifying a legal document. How you feel now is a poor indication of how you will perform in the air.

Equally important, the odds are that the problem is resolvable. Also, on the FAA 8500-8 form you declare, in no uncertain terms, that you have answered the questions factually, to the best of your knowledge. You sign your name to that fact. The penalties for falsification are severe: a maximum $250,000 fine and up to five years in jail—or both. For your own sake, the next time you fill out 8500-8, reread it carefully.

Remember, should there be any reason for the FAA to review your medical files, such as after a minor incident while flying, any known medical problem that you "overlooked" could be reason enough to end your career. The medical problem you were hiding could have been insignificant, but the fact that you falsified a legal document and deceived the FAA is enough to jeopardize your medical certification, your airman's flying license, and your career. Additionally, if you have knowingly deceived the FAA (or lied on any official legal form), then an insurance company may not recognize your claim. In other words, if you were injured or killed in an airplane crash, an insurance company may not pay you or your family any money that is entitled to you because you were less then honest on a form! The odds are that somewhere, sometime, your medical application form will be challenged for any number of reasons.

The Examination

After filling out your portion of Form 8500-8, you are now subjected to various tests and the physical exam.

Your vision should be tested in one of two ways: reading a chart twenty feet away in a well-lighted area or using an apparatus that, through the use of mirrors, duplicates the conditions of near and distant objects.

An audiogram should always be performed. The old whispered voice test used to determine hearing ability is grossly inaccurate. The new "voice" or "conversational" test is more realistic (see FAR 67.105 in Appendix I) but still tells you little about the magnitude of any hearing loss. One objective of a hearing test is to determine an unknown hearing loss before it becomes disqualifying. Corrective action may be taken to prevent further hearing loss and to save your hearing as well as your career. Trying to get by with the voice test is, in my opinion, foolish and similar to cramming for an exam just to get by, even though the material in the exam is important.

A urine specimen is tested for the presence of sugar, which could signify diabetes or the tendency toward it, and albumin, which might indicate kidney disease.

Your blood pressure and pulse are taken. Note that the FAA requests a sitting blood pressure and only a resting pulse. The older Form 8500-8 accepted blood pressure taken while lying down and required exercise pulses.

The physical examination is done by the AME. Contrary to some opinions the examination should be the same for all classes of medical certification. The difference between first-, second-, and third-class certificates is not the type of physical given but the stringency of the criteria and medical standards that must be met (which may include a few extra tests such as an ECG) by each pilot applicant. However, the AME may be as critical with the evaluation as he or she feels is necessary for the type of flying to be done.

Another important point is that the FAA medical evaluation does not check for every health problem. Only basic screening tests are done to rule out the more significant problems. Medical history is still the most important part of any exam, but it is often not shared with the AME. Unless there is a reasonable cause for additional information, there is no testing, for example, for how you think or react, which is a major consideration of how age or a medical disorder affects the brain. A good case in point is the widely known FAA denial of a famous air show aerobatic pilot in the early 1990s. He passed the initial FAA medical standards, but a reasonable case was made that he could be mentally impaired. Therefore, additional testing was done, and the impairment was confirmed and became a part of the record. However, the press chose not to tell the whole story during the earlier stages of the appeal process, and the impression was that the FAA was being unfair. Often, alcoholism, a psychosis, kidney stones, ulcers, and many other conditions won't be picked up on the FAA medical exam. Therefore, even if you pass the FAA exam, you still may have a disqualifying medical condition.

The AME, therefore, becomes a key player in certification. The more knowledgeable an AME is about flying and the bureaucracy of the FAA, the more that AME can be a true asset to you. An AME who is a "white knuckler" when it comes to flying could be overly critical. One who has no interest in flying or in working with the FAA may take the whole medical evaluation process for granted and not realize the importance of the exam.

Pilots may have a false sense of security when their AME is someone who is not adequately familiar with the FAA certification process or how a health problem affects safe flying. A single battery of blood tests does not prove you are in good health unless the results are considered along with the rest of an exam. A nonaeromedical doctor may think your condition is safe when, in fact, it may not be to the FAA. The statement by a doctor that "You'll never fly again" is no less misleading than "I see no reason why you can't fly."

Ideally, the AME should be a pilot, should be familiar with the requirements and expectations of FAA protocol, and should desire to assist you in your certification beyond the initial medical exam.

The Usual Outcome of the Examination

After the exam, the AME reviews all the data obtained from your medical history, the testing procedures, and the examination. He or she will then deter-

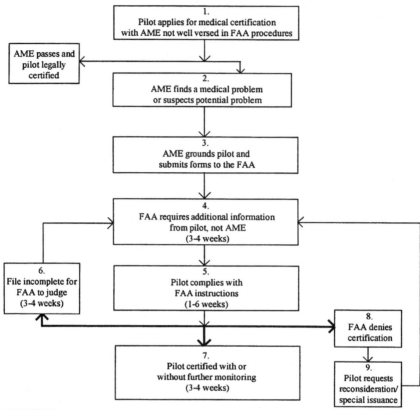

COMMENTS:
1. Many AMEs are not highly knowledgeable regarding expeditious handling of problem certification.
2. Often, the AME does not tell the pilot the significance of findings, letting the FAA be the "bad guy" and inform the pilot he/she is grounded.
3. Often the AME prematurely submits an inc incomplete report to the FAA.
4. The FAA requires additional medical information to reconsider a pilot's fitness to fly.
5. The pilot often is left on his/her own to work with specialists and handle the additional paperwork required by the FAA.
6. Because of misunderstandings concerning the intent of further evaluation and requirements, the FAA requests further data and the pilot is back to #4.
7. The pilot is finally certified, but not after many unnecessary delays.
8. By this point, the pilot often is trying to coordinate and achieve cooperation from three entities, the original AME, any specialists who have entered the proceedings, and the FAA.
9. The pilot can request reconsideration or special issuance reviews as often as he/she wants, as long as something new is presented and/or time has passed.

The key to why there is an improperly handled certification sequence is not knowing and properly anticipating what the FAA needs in advance of its requests. Tremendous amounts of time can be lost by waiting for the FAA to respond to previous paperwork submission, only to learn that more paperwork is necessary. Incomplete paperwork or failure to comply with the FAA's requests accounts for the majority of all denials and delays.

Improperly managed certification sequence

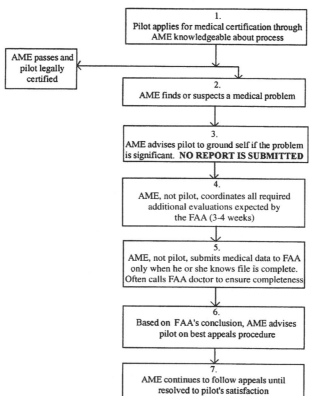

```
┌─────────────────────────────────┐
│              1.                 │
│ Pilot applies for medical       │
│ certification through           │
│ AME knowledgeable about process │
└─────────────────────────────────┘
```

AME passes and pilot legally certified

```
┌─────────────────────────────────┐
│              2.                 │
│ AME finds or suspects a         │
│ medical problem                 │
└─────────────────────────────────┘

┌─────────────────────────────────┐
│              3.                 │
│ AME advises pilot to ground     │
│ self if the problem             │
│ is significant. NO REPORT IS    │
│ SUBMITTED                       │
└─────────────────────────────────┘

┌─────────────────────────────────┐
│              4.                 │
│ AME, not pilot, coordinates     │
│ all required additional         │
│ evaluations expected by         │
│ the FAA (3-4 weeks)             │
└─────────────────────────────────┘

┌─────────────────────────────────┐
│              5.                 │
│ AME, not pilot, submits         │
│ medical data to FAA only when   │
│ he or she knows file is         │
│ complete. Often calls FAA       │
│ doctor to ensure completeness   │
└─────────────────────────────────┘

┌─────────────────────────────────┐
│              6.                 │
│ Based on FAA's conclusion,      │
│ AME advises pilot on best       │
│ appeals procedure               │
└─────────────────────────────────┘

┌─────────────────────────────────┐
│              7.                 │
│ AME continues to follow         │
│ appeals until resolved to       │
│ pilot's satisfaction            │
└─────────────────────────────────┘
```

COMMENTS:

1. This is the key to success of control: the AME is knowledgeable in the certification process and aviation medicine and is experienced in working with the FAA in protecting the fit to fly pilot.
2. The AME will try to anticipate, by using the AME's guide, potential problems that can be resolved with the FAA.
3. This is the second key to success: no report is made to the FAA until both the AME and pilot are satisfied with the file. If the pilot's condition is not significant, the pilot continues to fly.
4. The AME can make appointments with a specialist and explain the FAA expectations to that doctor.
5. The AME submits the entire file to the FAA, with a cover letter, rather than making the FAA the coordinator of the varied medical reports. The AME may call an FAA doctor to clarify what additional information is needed, if any.
6. If the FAA still does not certify, then the AME can determine what courses of action to follow by discussing the file with FAA doctors.
7. The AME should commit himself/herself to the pilot to assist the pilot in getting through the entire appeals, reconsideration, and special issuance process and explain why such actions are necessary.

Properly managed certification sequence

mine if you have any disqualifying conditions as defined in the *Guide for Aviation Medical Examiners* (see Appendix II). This guide is a comprehensive review and interpretation of the medical regulations and what the FAA expects to be submitted along with the application when the standards are not met. If there are no problems noted, the AME will certify you. Basically, the AME need only obtain the minimum data, make a decision to certify or not certify, and submit Form 8500-8 to the FAA for final judgment. The FAA then determines if it can confirm the issuance of your certificate with or without a waiver or limitation. If not, the FAA will request additional information from the pilot.

That request can sound rather intimidating. You might read between the lines of the letter and assume you are grounded. That is not the case unless the FAA asks you to return your certificate. It will often state that it is unable to establish your certifiability without additional information, but that doesn't mean you can't fly. (If the FAA is grounding you, the letter will usually be certified.) The time for compliance also causes unnecessary concern. If you can't meet the FAA's deadline, ask your AME to request an extension or do it yourself by phone or letter. In any case, unless the letter states otherwise, you can go on flying—but don't forget that the FAA is expecting a response. It won't forget!

There is one situation that warrants comment: an AME may choose not to mention a disqualifying condition to the pilot. In this situation, the pilot leaves the office assuming that all is OK, only to get a letter several weeks or months later stating that there is, in fact, a potential abnormality requiring more data before certification. An equally scary situation is when an AME says, "you'll never fly again," without any suggestions about what the pilot can do to regain certification. No denial is final unless you accept it as final—the FAA will always reconsider your application if you can give it additional proof that you aren't a risk.

I feel there are few circumstances, if any, in which the AME cannot anticipate the FAA's response before Form 8500-8 is submitted. The AME who elects not to tell you that you may be grounded may not want to be the "bad guy"; however, passing the buck to the FAA results in unnecessary delays. The FAA even encourages AMEs to do this in order to maintain the AME's respectability and the trust of the rest of the pilot group and to keep the AME from making decisions that aren't appropriate. The FAA assumes, though, that this AME has performed a good evaluation and has at least informed the pilot of what to expect, even if the doctor doesn't want to get involved. If this additional evaluation isn't performed, the pilot must wait for the FAA's instructions. Those same instructions are in the AME's guidebook.

Know your AME's philosophy about certification beforehand. The key question to be asked of any examining AME involved in your certification is "What does the AME do if he or she finds something wrong?" The AME's response is an indication of his or her knowledge of you, your career, and the FAA plus the AME's willingness to work with you on your behalf.

Instead of ignoring the problem, the AME may give you some indication of your situation by saying, "I don't think you have a disqualifying problem and in my opinion the FAA should certify you, but the book says that I can't certify you because of x result. I'll have to send everything in to the FAA and let them decide. Sorry." The AME will not issue the certificate at that time; you must wait until the FAA gets around to passing judgment or requesting more data and everyone gets defensive. You're stuck in the middle again.

Once Form 8500-8 is sent from the AME's office to the FAA, either by mail or electronically through the AMCS, the wheels of the bureaucracy begin their sluggish turning. The pass the buck philosophy may be common, but there is a better way. You obviously aren't qualified to play doctor, but if you know the system and how it can work, you will have better control of your future and will even be able to assist your AME should you develop a problem in your medical certification.

A BETTER OUTCOME TO THE CERTIFICATION PROCESS

Let's go back to that place in the certification process where the AME has finished the evaluation and is ready to lay judgment on you and to submit Form 8500-8 to Oklahoma City. Again, if all is OK, that's the end of the process until the next exam. If, however, some abnormality is found, whether proven or suspected, the following sequence of events could take place, and many of the "not normals" could be resolved quickly by competent hands. The following are ways the AME and the FAA can keep you flying, even with less than perfect results from a physical exam.

Limitations

If the AME finds a condition that is not perfect, he or she has the authority to issue you a certificate provided you adhere to certain limitations. The most common example is poor distant vision, which requires glasses or contact lenses to correct. The limitation, which is written on the front of your medical certificate in the "Limitations" block, would then read, "Holder shall wear (or 'possess' in the case of poor near vision) lenses that correct for distant vision while exercising the privileges of his airman's certificate." The limitation "Not valid for night flight or by color signal control" is used for color deficient pilots who cannot get a waiver or SODA (Statement of Demonstrated Ability).

To determine how you are to fly with a defect, limitations may be placed on the certificate after further evaluation by authorities; these are not necessarily medical authorities (for example, check pilots might be authorized to

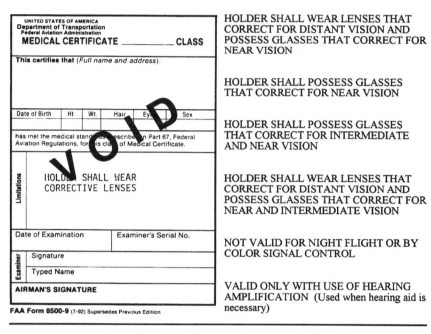

UNITED STATES OF AMERICA
Department of Transportation
Federal Aviation Administration
MEDICAL CERTIFICATE _____ **CLASS**

This certifies that (*Full name and address*):

| Date of Birth | Ht | Wt. | Hair | Eyes | Sex |

has met the medical standards prescribed in Part 67, Federal Aviation Regulations, for this class of Medical Certificate.

Limitations
HOLDER SHALL WEAR CORRECTIVE LENSES

| Date of Examination | Examiner's Serial No. |

Examiner
Signature
Typed Name

AIRMAN'S SIGNATURE

FAA Form 8500-9 (7-92) Supersedes Previous Edition

HOLDER SHALL WEAR LENSES THAT CORRECT FOR DISTANT VISION AND POSSESS GLASSES THAT CORRECT FOR NEAR VISION

HOLDER SHALL POSSESS GLASSES THAT CORRECT FOR NEAR VISION

HOLDER SHALL POSSESS GLASSES THAT CORRECT FOR INTERMEDIATE AND NEAR VISION

HOLDER SHALL WEAR LENSES THAT CORRECT FOR DISTANT VISION AND POSSESS GLASSES THAT CORRECT FOR NEAR AND INTERMEDIATE VISION

NOT VALID FOR NIGHT FLIGHT OR BY COLOR SIGNAL CONTROL

VALID ONLY WITH USE OF HEARING AMPLIFICATION (Used when hearing aid is necessary)

Examples of limitations as stated on a medical certificate

evaluate an in-flight pilot with a medical or physical problem). Then, after being reviewed by the FAA, you will be certified with an appropriate limitation (if necessary) and allowed to fly. Sometimes a waiver or SODA will be issued, and nothing will be printed on your certificate. The limitation is a part of your certificate, and you must be able to prove you are following its conditions when flying.

In addition to medical limitations there are operational limitations whereby the FAA can limit the functions of the pilot to certain crew positions (e.g., "duties not to include pilot in command" or "valid for flight engineer only"). The FAA used to be able to limit a first-class medical certificate to certain crew positions, but courts have concluded that the FAA does not have this authority. The rules allow for such limitations only for second- and third-class medical certificates.

Medical Waivers and Statements of Demonstrated Ability (SODAs)

Prior to the 1996 amendments, there was some confusion about SODAs, medical waivers, and special issuances. The SODA and waiver are meant to allow you to fly even though you do not meet the specific medical standards stated in the regulations. The 1996 changes state that a SODA is issued when the pilot can demonstrate the ability to fly safely with some medical or physical impairment or disability, such as having only one eye, a deficient color vision, or an amputation. A waiver is intended for a condition that doesn't meet the stated standards but is considered an acceptable risk after further testing and review. Getting medically certified for a major medical problem (such as one of the mandatory denied conditions) through special issuance is now called an "authorization."

If your medical condition is not necessarily detrimental to safe flying, even though it could be cause for a denial, the FAA (not the AME) may grant a SODA or a waiver. You must prove that the presence of the problem does not interfere with safe flying and that you will not become impaired months after the certification is issued. Prior to the 1996 medical standards revision, the SODA was most commonly used in cases of very poor uncorrected distant vision (worse that 20/100 for first class). However, there is no longer an uncorrected vision standard; you still have to have the limitation requiring you to wear and/or possess glasses but the SODA is no longer needed for this deficiency. Medical conditions such as hearing not being in the acceptable limits as stated in the AME guide and a color vision deficiency still need the SODA.

A SODA or waiver differs from a limitation in that the medical criteria can be foregone if it can be proven that the medical condition or physical disability does not interfere with safe flying. A pilot does this by actually demonstrating flying abilities to other examiners (again, not necessarily doctors). A limitation, on the other hand, is what the pilot must do, such as wear glasses, to be properly "equipped" to fly and meet regulations (see page 48).

With a limitation, the deficiency must be corrected by some method while flying. With a SODA, the pilot's ability and experience compensate for the deficiency. A SODA allows pilots to prove that their condition is not risky, even though they technically don't meet the letter of the FAA standards or the conditions explained in the AME's guide.

A SODA is not a black mark on your record. It is actually protection granted by the FAA against being unnecessarily grounded by an AME. In fact, the pilot is encouraged to get a SODA on file with the FAA to preclude an unnecessary delay in certification from an AME who doesn't know the pilot or isn't sure what to do with the pilot's test results.

A SODA is not issued if you have a condition that is medically disqualifying and that could interfere with safe flying in the form of an unexpected and sudden impairment, incapacitation, or distraction. In these cases, a medical waiver is issued, usually in the form of a letter. This is not a separate paper certificate like the SODA, which must be carried with you along with your other certificates. Some examples of situations requiring a medical waiver include blood pressure that is too high, a kidney stone, or ulcers. For these conditions,

MEDICAL CERTIFICATE ___SECOND___ CLASS

UNITED STATES OF AMERICA
DEPARTMENT OF TRANSPORTATION
FEDERAL AVIATION ADMINISTRATION

THIS CERTIFIES THAT (Full name and address)

John Q. Public
800 Independence Avenue, S.W.
Washington, D.C. 20590

DATE OF BIRTH	HEIGHT	WEIGHT	HAIR	EYES	SEX
6-5-22	5'11"	165	Brown	Blue	M.

has met the medical standards prescribed in Part 67, Federal Aviation Regulations for this class of Medical Certificate

LIMITATIONS

Must wear back brace while flying.

DATE OF EXAMINATION	EXAMINER'S SERIAL NO
May 3, 1970	0001-08-8

EXAMINER SIGNATURE *P. V. Siegel MD*

TYPED NAME P. V. Siegel, M.D.

AIRMAN'S SIGNATURE

FAA FORM 8500-9 (1-67) SUPERSEDES FAA FORM 1004-1

STATEMENT OF DEMONSTRATED ABILITY

UNITED STATES OF AMERICA
DEPARTMENT OF TRANSPORTATION
FEDERAL AVIATION ADMINISTRATION

This form cannot be used in lieu of a medical certificate; it should be attached to your medical certificate.

AIRMAN'S NAME AND ADDRESS

John Q. Public
800 Independence Ave., S.W.
Washington, D.C. 20590

CLASS OF MEDICAL CERTIFICATE AUTHORIZED	WAIVER SERIAL NO.						
SECOND CLASS	3	8	W	5	7	0	2	5

LIMITATIONS

Must wear back brace while flying.

PHYSICAL DEFECTS

Lumbosacral strain

BASIS OF ISSUANCE

[ ] OPERATIONAL EXPERIENCE   [ ] SPECIAL PRACTICAL TEST   [X] SPECIAL FLIGHT TEST

[X] Special Medical Examination

FOR THE FEDERAL AIR SURGEON

DATE May 3, 1970

SIGNATURE (TO BE SIGNED IN INK)

P. V. Siegel MD

NAME AND TITLE (TO BE TYPED)
P. V. SIEGEL, M.D.
FEDERAL AIR SURGEON

FAA Form 8500-18 (12-69) FORMERLY FAA FORM 770

MEDICAL CERTIFICATE ___THIRD___ CLASS

UNITED STATES OF AMERICA
DEPARTMENT OF TRANSPORTATION
FEDERAL AVIATION ADMINISTRATION

THIS CERTIFIES THAT (Full name and address)

SPECIMEN COPY

DATE OF BIRTH	HEIGHT	WEIGHT	HAIR	EYES	SEX
7-7-42	6'1"	175	Br.	Br.	M.

has met the medical standards prescribed in Part 67, Federal Aviation Regulations for this class of Medical Certificate

LIMITATIONS

Holder shall wear contact lens (left eye) and shall possess correcting glasses for near vision while exercising the privileges of his airman certificate.

DATE OF EXAMINATION	EXAMINER'S SERIAL NO
May 3, 1970	0001-08-8

EXAMINER SIGNATURE *P. V. Siegel MD*

TYPED NAME P. V. Siegel, M.D.

AIRMAN'S SIGNATURE

FAA FORM 8500-9 (1-67) SUPERSEDES FAA FORM 1004-1

STATEMENT OF DEMONSTRATED ABILITY

UNITED STATES OF AMERICA
DEPARTMENT OF TRANSPORTATION
FEDERAL AVIATION ADMINISTRATION

This form cannot be used in lieu of a medical certificate; it should be attached to your medical certificate.

AIRMAN'S NAME AND ADDRESS

SPECIMEN COPY

CLASS OF MEDICAL CERTIFICATE AUTHORIZED	WAIVER SERIAL NO.						
THIRD CLASS	4	8	G	5	7	0	3	5

LIMITATIONS Holder shall wear contact lens (left eye) and shall possess correcting glasses for near vision while exercising the privileges of his airman certificate.

PHYSICAL DEFECTS Distant visual acuity:
(R: 20/20) L: Aphakic, corr 20/20 w/contact lens

BASIS OF ISSUANCE

[X] OPERATIONAL EXPERIENCE   [ ] SPECIAL PRACTICAL TEST   [ ] SPECIAL FLIGHT TEST

[X] Special Medical Evaluation

FOR THE FEDERAL AIR SURGEON

DATE May 3, 1970

SIGNATURE (TO BE SIGNED IN INK)

P. V. Siegel MD

NAME AND TITLE (TO BE TYPED)
P. V. SIEGEL, M.D.
FEDERAL AIR SURGEON

FAA Form 8500-18 (12-69) FORMERLY FAA FORM 770

Medical certificates with limitations and Statements of Demonstrated Ability the FAA passes judgment based on the additional medical data provided by you and your doctors. (These conditions will be described later in the chapter.)

You are certified to fly if the added medical data proves you are an acceptable risk even though your medical condition could potentially cause a problem. Each case is evaluated on its own merits and risk factors. Your AME may need to be encouraged to help more than usual.

Until now we have been discussing less serious medical conditions, conditions that could be resolved through additional testing and through the AME working with the doctors in Oklahoma City to determine what action is necessary. Yet we are all aware of unnecessarily long delays for minor problems such as high blood pressure when a waiver should have been easily and quickly obtained.

Although getting supplemental data is your responsibility, your AME should know what needs to be done and should be able to expedite the action for you. After all, that's what you are paying the AME to do, and that's what the FAA expects. If your AME doesn't know what to do because the AME's guide is unclear for your situation, either you or your AME can simply call Oklahoma City or the Regional Flight Surgeon in your area for instructions.

There can be complete confidentiality while you are getting guidance on the next step. Just keep in mind FAR 61.53. Don't fly if you are not well so that you or your AME won't have to report anything to the FAA until everything is in order.

Conditions That Are Disqualifying

Even though more authority is being given to AMEs, there are conditions that, generally, your AME has no authority to judge and must turn over to the FAA for consideration. Several conditions (discussed in Chapter 2) are "mandatory" denials: that is, the regulations make no exceptions, and even the Federal Air Surgeon has no choice but to deny you initially. The appeal process (special issuance) for these cases will be discussed later. What we will discuss now is how the other disqualifying conditions can be certified—those other less serious but numerous conditions listed in the AME's guide. Keep in mind that the formal medical standards (Part 67) are not specific for each medical disorder. Most will be further defined in the AME's guide.

Although less serious than the mandatory denials, these are the conditions that cause the most problems in getting certified, create the most misunderstanding, and result in the greatest waste of time if not properly handled. If properly handled by you and your AME, these cases should be resolved in a matter of a few weeks.

At this point, I want to discuss a little known part of the medical regulations, namely paragraph 67.401, "special issuance of medical certificates" (the old 67.19). It's worth reading. This is a particularly important paragraph because it gives the Federal Air Surgeon the authority to certify essentially every medical problem, even the mandatory denials, if it can be proven with factual medical data that the pilot is safe to fly in the type of aircraft and position for which the pilot is applying. Once again, if you can prove that your medical disorder is an acceptable risk now and in the next six to twelve months, then no matter what the problem is the Federal Air Surgeon can consider certifying you.

In years past, the Federal Air Surgeon could not certify a pilot with disqualifying conditions, even if it could be shown that the pilot was safe to fly. Prior to 1982, there was an "exemption process." That is, since the Federal Air Surgeon couldn't certify a medically safe pilot, a grant of exemption (an administrative action) from the regulations was issued—an exemption not from the restrictions of the medical problem but from the stipulations of the old Part 67. After getting around the restrictions through an exemption, the FAA could consider the pilot's medical status. This took six to twelve months or more, mainly due to the administrative requirements inherent in the exemption process.

With the 1982 amendments, the Federal Air Surgeon was no longer restricted from certifying the old "nine mandatory disorders" that were part of the regulations prior to 1996. Today there are additional mandatory denials, but the process of Special Issuance remains in effect (Appendix I). Part 67.401 is self-explanatory, and it is the intent of this paragraph to be in the best interests of the pilot and safe flight. In any case, you will still need to provide the same medical information as described throughout the book. In other words, your responsibility to prove your fitness to fly hasn't changed. The intent now is that the Federal Air Surgeon has the authority to certify you for any disorders—if you are fit to fly.

Before I get into details, let me once again state what I believe are acceptable methods of certification if everyone respects the other's responsibilities and obligations. If you feel that there is any doubt that your medical condition is going to interfere with safe flying—don't fly. Ground yourself. The FAA doesn't need to know about your health until you are ready to go back to flying. It's not illegal to be sick as long as you don't fly! FAR 61.53 applies only if you fly.

Your chief concern is not the possibility of illness, it's what happens to you and your career and your FAA medical certificate when you and your "illness" are reported to the FAA. Your doctor should be able to tell you what is wrong, why it is incompatible with safe flying, and what needs to be done to make your condition acceptable to the FAA. The FAA wants only medically safe pilots at the controls—you don't have to be in perfect health! Even if the FAA does not certify you right away, you will be many steps ahead of the poor pilot who is an innocent victim of the pass the buck process.

In my judgment, if you are grounded, there is no need to immediately report your condition to the FAA until you have everything in order—provided you consult your AME and defer flying until approved by the FAA. The FAA must be allowed to review the accumulated medical data before returning you to flying status. By compiling all the required data in one file and submitting it to the FAA along with your certificate application you avoid getting into the red tape of the bureaucracy, and you have a better chance of getting back to flying.

There will be those who will ask, "What about the sick pilot who continues to fly?" When discussing how the process can work, I am not talking about the irresponsible pilot who doesn't trust anyone. Some even fly without certification, often bragging that they don't need it! These pilots are a menace to colleagues and the public, and I worry more about the pilots' sense of responsibility, logic, and attitude than their medical condition. There is enough redundancy in professional flying that peers will be able to cover for a pilot if he or she does become seriously ill while flying. But the fact remains that the pilot is in violation of the FARs. In the future, licensed recreational pilots (not private pilots) may be able to medically certify themselves. What the conditions and process will be remains to be seen.

In the interests of safety and shared liability, an irresponsible pilot should be reported to someone, maybe to the pilot's peers first, but certainly to someone who can keep the pilot from endangering him- or herself and others. There is always someone that can be informed of this situation, even if the pilot may be unaware of his or her potential violation. The added concern is the example it sets—if this person can get away with abusing the privilege to fly, then others can reason that it's OK.

This complacent attitude hurts the credibility of those professionals who want to help a responsible pilot return to flying status. Irresponsible pilots are in the minority, but they are still a part of our system. I feel that we must respect responsible pilots who do not want to fly because they are ill. Their return to flying status should be handled by a doctor who knows how to help. That should be an AME!

There are also those who would criticize this approach by saying that the FAA requires that it be informed right away to keep the irresponsible pilot from flying. This is a valid consideration. That is why the FAA encourages (not demands) the AME to report significantly sick pilots who are flying. The FAA knows that the majority of professional civilian pilots lack adequate medical monitoring and supervision, thus necessitating immediate disclosure when something is discovered. Therefore, as discussed earlier, the lack of support of some of the AMEs has led the FAA to be more "possessive" of its responsibility to enforce the regulations to protect the public from the minority of pilots who would abuse the privilege of flying. This is perceived by many pilots and aviation organizations as being overly restrictive.

There is also the inference that because no accidents are officially caused by the medical problems identified by the FAA there is no need for even the medical exam. The fault with that reasoning is that a medical problem can cause impairment, distraction, poor decision making, and reduced reaction time, but these are rarely cited as causative factors in an accident report.

Still, if you are not flying while you are being further evaluated and you remain self-grounded until the FAA acts on the medical data, you are not breaking any rules. More important is the fact that you remain in control of your future instead of placing it entirely in the hands of the FAA. If your AME is unable or unwilling "to pick up the ball," then you have to rely on the FAA to tell you what to do. As mentioned before, it is your responsibility to seek the added data for certification; it's not the responsibility of the AME or the FAA (remember that all correspondence from the FAA is mailed to you and not the AME). But you don't have to do it alone or wait for the FAA to respond. Tell your AME to hold your file until either you or the AME calls the FAA for guidance.

But you shouldn't have to tell the AME this. Every AME has the *Guide for Aviation Medical Examiners* (see Appendix II) and the information to help you meet FAA expectations. The AME may choose not to get involved, however, and then it is in your hands to find another AME or check with the FAA.

If you and your AME feel that you are healthy enough to fly while the additional evaluation is going on, have your AME call the FAA for guidance and possibly for permission to continue flying while tests are being done. Initially, no names need to be mentioned. The FAA may approve your request if there is no compromise to safety. If it says no, don't fly. The FAA still does not need to know who you are if you respect FAR 61.53, and you can go on to the next step.

On the back of the 8500-8 form, item 62 is where the AME recommends what course of action should be taken as a result of the exam. In most cases of potential denials, the "deferred" box should be checked, signifying that, although you may have a disqualifying condition according to the regulations, there could be added data to prove that you are not a safety risk. If the AME elects to pass the buck, he or she will check this box but not add any data. By doing this, the AME instructs the FAA to tell you what the next step is. The AME should know this next step and should provide additional, explanatory data along with Form 8500-8.

Checking the "denied" box could complicate the ease of recertification, although the FAA will always reopen your file to consider new information. The FAA will write you, stating the AME's decision along with the FAA's, which could include medical certification, a denial, or a request for more information. Another reason to ask that a denial be deferred to the FAA is that future applications for medical certification will ask if you have ever been denied (item 13). Again, this isn't a major roadblock, but it would be better if you didn't have to answer yes, especially if your problem is not significant and ultimately certifiable.

There are cases in which it is obvious to the AME that applicants should not fly or in which the applicants know they are grounded or even want to be grounded. Then the AME sends a letter of denial to the applicant, with a copy to the FAA. The FAA will review the data submitted by the AME and, if it concurs, will confirm the denial with a similar letter. This official denial is important so that professional pilots can prove their "medical retirement" and justify their claim to their disability insurance carriers. Instructions are still given to grounded pilots for further appeal procedures.

Attention CFIs: be sure to instruct your new students to get their medical certificate as soon as they begin instruction. I have seen too many disappointed and angry pilots who were scheduled to solo and then had a problem found at their exam. Even if the students are ultimately certified, they won't be in time for the solo.

RECERTIFICATION FOR DENIED CONDITIONS

More medical data will be required for the FAA to make a decision about possible recertification of a disqualifying medical condition. With adequate documentation of additional tests and data that prove that the "abnormal" condition is not significant and would not jeopardize the safety of flying, most pilots eventually can be certified. It's essential to recognize that only 0.1 percent of all applications end up being denied, so the odds are with you. Remember, although instructions for recertification are intended for your doctor, you are the one to whom they will be sent. The FAA can't tell you what doctor to see, but your AME can suggest someone, not necessarily an AME, and even help set up appointments.

These protocols (see pages 54-61) delineate what the FAA requires—strictly requires. These instructions are a part of the AME's guide, so an AME shouldn't tell you that he or she doesn't know what the FAA will want.

You would think that these specifications are straightforward, but failure to follow these instructions is one of the areas where the recertification process gets held up, and you get caught in the middle. Some doctors do not agree with the FAA's instructions for evaluating a medical disorder and would rather fight the system than provide the required data. The FAA has a reason for wanting certain tests, reasons that many nonaviation doctors don't understand or respect. A doctor's opinion as to what is necessary and not necessary will only delay the process until that doctor complies.

Some doctors may be correct in thinking the way they do, but whether or not their medical community commonly uses a specified test is not important. What is important is that the FAA requires it. Usually, if something is not per-

FAA SPECIFICATIONS FOR PSYCHIATRIC AND PSYCHOLOGICAL EVALUATIONS

I. If not previously submitted, all records are required covering prior psychiatric hospitalizations and/or other periods of observation or treatment. These records must be in sufficient detail to permit a clear evaluation of the nature and extent of any previous mental disorders.

II. A report by a qualified psychiatrist is required. (A qualified psychiatrist is preferably one who has been certified by the American Board of Psychiatry and Neurology, or one who has a background equivalent for Board certifications.) The applicant's personal physician is often a good source for such a referral.

The examination must be of recent date, and the report should be in sufficient detail and depth to permit an accurate evaluation of the petitioner's interval history, and his/her current psychiatric status. The usual elements of an evaluation such as past history, family history, and current mental status should be included as well.

III. A report is also required by a qualified clinical psychologist who is experienced in administering such tests. (A qualified psychologist is preferably one with a state license or certification with a Ph.D. in Clinical Psychology, or is listed in the National Register of Health Service Providers in Psychology.) The applicant may contact the local psychological association for a referral.

The report (including a copy of the test protocols) should contain a detailed psychological evaluation based on a battery of psychological tests. Such a battery should include: (1) the complete Wechsler Adult Intelligence Scale-Revised (WAIS-R), (2) the Minnesota Multiphasic Personality Inventory (MMPI-2/MMPI), and as considered appropriate by the practitioner, any three *or more* of the remaining tests or their equivalents:

a. A cognitive function screening test such as the Trails Making Test, Category Test (Booklet or Machine), or a memory scale (Wechsler Memory Scale, California Verbal Learning Test, Rey Auditory Verbal Learning Test).

b. A projective test such as the Rorschach or Sentence Completion.

c. A personality inventory test such as the NEO-R, the Personality Assessment Inventory, the Millon Clinical Multiaxial Inventory (MCMI).

d. A symptom screening test such as the Beck or Hamilton for depression, or the MAST for Alcoholism.

The evaluating psychologist should select the particular tests based upon his or her experience, considering the particular issues involved.

[Revised January 22, 1996, from Form 8500-26]

FAA specifications for reconsideration and special issuance of specific medical disorders

SPECIFICATIONS FOR PSYCHIATRIC AND PSYCHOLOGICAL EVALUATIONS IN CASES INVOLVING SUBSTANCE ABUSE/DEPENDENCE

When a history of substance abuse/dependence is in question in an applicant for medical certification, it is the responsibility of the Office of Aviation Medicine to determine whether a problem does exist; and if it does, whether there is satisfactory evidence of recovery. To this end, both current psychiatric and psychological evaluations are required, as well as all records of observation and treatment. The psychiatrist and psychologist should submit separate reports.

A report by a qualified psychiatrist is required. It is recommended that the psychiatric evaluation be conducted by a psychiatrist experienced in the diagnosis and treatment of all types of addiction. All pertinent medical records and professional reports should be made available to the psychiatrist prior to the preparation of the report. The usual elements of an evaluation, such as past history, family history, and current mental status should be included as well.

Evidence pertaining to the quality of recovery should also be included in the psychiatrist's report. An opinion as to whether there is history of addiction should be based upon the following definition, contained in the Federal Aviation Regulations. [Note: Check with the 1996 revision of the medical standards, which includes drug abuse as well as dependence.]

ALCOHOLISM: As used in this section, "alcoholism" means a condition in which a person's intake of alcohol has been great enough to damage his or her physical health or personal or social functioning, or when alcohol has become a prerequisite to normal functioning.

DRUG DEPENDENCE: As used in the section, "drug dependence" means a condition in which a person is addicted to or dependent on drugs other than alcohol, tobacco, or ordinary caffeine-containing beverages, as evidenced by habitual use or a clear sense of need for the drug.

[Note: The remainder of these specifications are the same as noted above in the section on general psychiatric conditions. These specifications are current with the 1996 FARs revisions.]

[Revised February 10, 1995]

SPECIFICATIONS FOR NEUROLOGICAL EVALUATION

I. If not previously submitted, all records are required covering prior hospitalizations and/or other periods of observation and treatment. These records must be in sufficient detail to permit a clear evaluation of the nature and extent of any previous neurologic disorder. Medical release forms are enclosed for you to complete and send to the physicians and/or hospitals which hold your records. You should request that copies of your records be mailed directly to this address. Please date and sign the release forms and return them to us for our records. An envelope is provided for this purpose.

[Note: This specification is not unique to this disorder; it is a condition for all additional information sent to the FAA. It is preferred that every report be submitted in one file, preferably by an AME who can determine if the file is complete. However, should you choose to seek reconsideration on your own, then you must ensure the FAA has the release forms in its file for future reports.]

II. A report by a qualified neurologist is required. (A "qualified" neurologist is preferably one who has been certified by the American Board of Psychiatry and Neurology or by the American Board of Neurological Surgery, or one who has the background equivalent for Board certification. The applicant's personal physician is often a good source for such a referral.)

The neurologist's report must supply the following:

1. Detailed report of a recent neurological examination.

2. Additional information as stated in the AME's guide, depending on the disorder.

SPECIFICATIONS FOR INITIAL EVALUATION OF
ABNORMAL CARBOHYDRATE METABOLISM

[Note: "Abnormal carbohydrate metabolism" refers to sugar found in the urine during any FAA medical exam or elevated blood sugar found in any other exam. Diabetes is the first consideration that must be ruled out even though other conditions can cause these findings. If diabetes is diagnosed, then refer to the standards in Appendixes II and III.]

The condition should be adequately controlled for at least three months.

I. Control is to be documented by determining, at least at monthly intervals, that the fasting blood sugar and glycosylated hemoglobin do not, in preponderance, exceed normal values.

II. There are no disqualifying medical or surgical complications, including cardiac disease, peripheral vascular disease, renal disease, neurological abnormalities, or ocular changes.

III. There is no history of significant hypoglycemic reactions or evidence of an unusual risk or tendency for such reactions.

IV. No beta-adrenergic blocking agents are being used by the applicant and the applicant's natural adrenergic response system is intact.

[Revised September 3, 1996]

CARDIOVASCULAR EVALUATION SPECIFICATIONS

[Note: For high blood pressure (hypertension), the following is generally a good start. However, some tests are not necessary, such as the exercise ECG. To help the AME expeditiously certify hypertension, check Appendix II for a more complete review of the FAA's expectations. Check with your AME as to specific current requirements for your medical problem.]

These specifications have been developed by the Federal Aviation Administration (FAA) to determine an applicant's eligibility for airman medical certification. Standardization of examination methods and reporting is essential to provide sufficient basis for making this determination and the prompt processing of applications. This cardiovascular evaluation, therefore, must be reported in sufficient detail to permit a clear and objective evaluation of the cardiovascular disorder(s) with emphasis on the degree of functional recovery and prognosis. Preferably, it should be performed by a specialist in internal medicine or cardiology and should be forwarded to the FAA immediately upon completion. Inadequate evaluation or reporting, or failure to promptly submit the report to the FAA, may delay the certification decision. As a minimum, the evaluation must include the following:

I. MEDICAL HISTORY. Particular reference would be given to cardiovascular abnormalities—cerebral, visceral, and/or peripheral. A statement must be included as to whether medications are currently or have been recently used, and if so, the type, purpose, dosage, duration of use, and other pertinent details must be given. A specific history of any anticoagulant drug therapy is required. In addition, any history of hypertension must be fully developed and if thiazide diuretics are being taken, values for serum potassium should be included on any important or unusual dietary programs.

II. FAMILY, PERSONAL, AND SOCIAL HISTORY. A statement of the ages and health status of parents and sibling is necessary; if deceased, age at death and cause should be included. Also, an indication of whether any near blood relative has had "heart attacks," hypertension, diabetes or known disorders of lipid metabolism must be provided. Smoking, drinking and recreational habits of the applicant are pertinent as well as whether a program of physical fitness is being maintained. Comments on the level of physical activities, function, limitations, occupation, and avocational pursuits are essential.

III. RECORDS OF PREVIOUS MEDICAL CARE. If not previously furnished to the FAA, a copy of pertinent hospital records as well as out-patient treatment records, with clinical data, X-ray and laboratory observations and originals or good copies of all electrographic (ECG) tracings, should be provided. Detailed reports of surgical procedures as well as cerebral and coronary arteriography and other major diagnostic studies are of prime importance.

IV. GENERAL PHYSICAL EXAMINATION. A brief description of any comment-worthy personal characteristics: height, weight, representative blood pressure reading in both arms, funduscopic examination of retinal arteries, condition of peripheral arteries (location, intensity, timing, and opinion as to significance) and other findings of consequence must be provided.

V. LABORATORY DATA. As a minimum, data must include actual values of:

a. Routine urinalysis and complete blood count.

b. Blood chemistries (values and normal ranges of the laboratory)
   1. Serum cholesterol and triglycerides after 12- to 16-hour fast.
   2. Fasting blood sugar. If the fasting blood sugar is elevated, include at least a 3-hour glucose tolerance test following glucose loading for 5 preceding days.

c. Electrocardiograms
   1. Resting tracing
   2. Bruce Protocol exercise stress test (maximal)
      a) Provide blood pressure determinations at rest at each stage of the exercise stress test and during the recovery periods
      b) Submit representative ECG tracings for the control, exercise, and recovery periods
      c) Obtain recovery ECG tracings until there is a return to the control configuration and/or until the control level of heart rate has been achieved

NOTE: If exercise stress testing is contraindicated, or if the person being tested is unable to perform a maximal effort test, please provide a full explanation.

d. If there is a history of valve replacement:
   1. Echocardiogram
   2. 24-hour Holtor Monitor Study
   3. Coagulation studies, if appropriate

e. If there is a history of pacemaker implantation:
   1. 24-hour Holtor Monitor Study
   2. Results of current pacemaker surveillance

[Form 8500-19, September 1996]

PROTOCOL FOR THE EVALUATION OF CORONARY HEART DISEASE

General requirements for the consideration for any class of airman medical certification:

1. A six-month recovery period shall elapse after the event (angina, infarction, bypass, surgery, or angioplasty) before consideration can be given for medical certification.

2. Copies of complete hospital/medical records pertaining to the angina, infarction, bypass surgery, or angioplasty, including admission/discharge summaries, operative reports, history and physical examination, daily progress reports, and all electrocardiogram (ECG) tracings and laboratory reports.

3. A current cardiovascular evaluation (Form 8500-19), preferably by a cardiologist or specialist in internal medicine. This evaluation must include an assessment of personal and family medical history, a clinical cardiac and general physical examination, and assessment and statement regarding the applicant's medications, functional capacity modifiable cardiovascular risk factors, motivations for any necessary change and prognosis for incapacitation during the certification period, fasting blood sugar, and a current blood lipid profile to include: total cholesterol, HDL, LDL, and triglycerides.

4. An ECG treadmill stress test must be performed no sooner than 6 months post event. All stress testing should achieve 100 percent of predicted maximal heart rate unless medically contraindicated or prevented by symptoms. Beta blockers and calcium channel blockers (specifically diltiazem and verapamil) or digitalis preparations should be discontinued for 48 hours prior to testing (if not contraindicated) in order to obtain maximum heart rate and only with consent of attending cardiologist. An applicant will be expected to demonstrate a minimum functional capacity equivalent to completion of stage 3 of a Bruce protocol and a double product of no less than 250×100. The work sheet with blood pressure/pulse recordings at various stages, interpretive report, and actual electrocardiographic tracings must be submitted.

Tracings must include a rhythm strip, a full 12-lead ECG recorded at rest (supine and standing) and during hyperventilation while standing, one or more times during each stage of exercise, at the end of each stage, at peak exercise, and every minute during recovery for at least five minutes or until the tracings return to baseline level. The interpretive report and work sheet must be submitted. Computer-generated sample cycle electrocardiographic tracings are *unacceptable* in lieu of the standard tracings and if submitted alone will result in deferment until this requirement is met.

A thallium exercise stress test may be required for consideration for any class, if clinically indicated or if the exercise stress test is unacceptable by any of the usual parameters. A SPECT-T1 is preferred with reinjection for redistribution imaging. (Subject to change as newer radionuclide substances are validated). The interpretive report and all scintigraphic images (in black and white monochrome on cut film if possible) must be submitted.

5. If cardiac catheterization and coronary angiography have been performed, all reports must be submitted, and films when requested, for review by the agency. Copies should be made of all films as a safeguard against loss.

In addition, for consideration for first or *unlimited second-class medical certification the following should be accomplished no sooner than 6 months post event.

6. Post event coronary angiography. Applications for first and unlimited second-class certification will not be considered without post event angiography. All reports and films must be submitted.

7. Operational Questionnaire Form 8500-20 must be completed. Airman should note if a lower class medical certificate is acceptable in the event of ineligibility for the class sought.

Applicants found qualified for an airman medical certificate shall be required to provide periodic, follow-up cardiovascular evaluations, including maximal stress testing. Additional diagnostic testing modalities, including radionuclide, may be required if indicated.

It is the responsibility of each applicant to provide the medical information required to determine his/her eligibility for airman medical certification.

All information shall be forwarded preferably in *one mailing* to:

Aeromedical Certification Division
Mike Monroney Aeronautical Center
Federal Aviation Administration
P.O. Box 26200
Oklahoma City, OK 73216

Attention: Special Issuance Branch, AAM-320

The use of the airman's full name, date of birth, and social security number on all correspondence and reports will aid the agency in locating the proper file

* An unlimited second-class medical certificate has no functional limitations. A limited second-class certificate with a functional limitation such as, "Not valid for carrying passengers for compensation or hire," "Not valid for pilot in command," "Valid only when serving as a pilot member of a fully qualified two-pilot crew," "Limited to flight engineer duties only," etc., may allow selected airmen to hold a second-class medical certificate when not eligible for an unlimited certificate.

[August 1996]

formed according to the protocol, the FAA will not consider it favorably. It seems much more realistic to me for my colleagues to swallow scientific pride, provide the FAA with what it wants, and get the job done swiftly. If your doctor feels that even more data would be in your best interest, great. But don't ignore the minimums set by the FAA, and tell your doctor not to ignore them.

Remember, the usual response by the FAA to an incomplete workup and file is, "Based on the information provided, we cannot certify your condition." Perhaps it could have been approved if all the data had been initially provided. It doesn't make sense to take shortcuts in the certification process when a career and medical certificate are at stake.

Many doctors who will be examining you to provide the additional data have the mistaken impression that they are expected to decide if you are fit and legal to fly. It's important to let them know that their role is only to provide the necessary information, without any opinions or judgment about whether or not you can fly. Some doctors with this impression may be overly restrictive or, on the other hand, minimize the significance of a medical problem. The statement often made in a report that "this medical problem should not interfere with flying and I see no reason why the patient shouldn't be certified" only confirms that doctor's lack of understanding.

Since it is the FAA's responsibility to make the decision, it is better for your doctor to stick to medical facts and not to comment on your fitness to fly—unless that doctor is familiar with the conditions of flying and FAA medical standards. Furthermore, your personal doctor will not be held liable if you are in an accident and he or she has done what is expected. So let your doctor know that his or her only role is to provide information, not decide if you can fly.

Another point that you and your AME must consider in choosing doctors is which are medically reputable and best qualified to provide data that will be accepted and respected by the FAA. This is truly a problem, and the individual pilot must rely on knowledgeable AMEs for advice. After all, most pilots do not frequent or need other doctors and specialists. The Airline Pilot's Association provides an aeromedical "coordinator" within its local union structure and an aeromedical physician at the national level who specializes in directing grounded pilots to appropriate consultants. (The union does not pick up the tab for the consultant's fee.) This is a valuable service to airline pilots who have no other resources. Air carriers with medical departments also can provide the services necessary to keep their pilots flying. Many local AMEs have a reputation for working with pilots to protect their medical certification. You just have to find out who those doctors are by asking around the hangar or FBO. Even the FAA knows of doctors who are cooperative.

So when the AME says, "I can't pass you because of *x* condition," the AME may tell you why *x* is disqualifying (unsafe for flying) until proven otherwise plus what needs to be done to satisfy the requirements of the FAA. Unfortunately, to adequately explain such a career-threatening situation to a pilot, who is understandably scared, takes a lot of time, time that most doctors don't have. This is another reason the AME might defer the decision concerning your certificate by sending the incomplete Form 8500-8 to the FAA. For now, let's assume that the AME is willing to act on your behalf and begins the process of obtaining the necessary additional data. The AME should be aware of what the FAA requires and open the door to consultants who appreciate what needs to be done. Ever try to get an appointment with a specialist as a new patient? It takes weeks or months!

Let's use an example to clarify the order of events so far. Your AME finds that your blood pressure is consistently too high. The AME explains the aeromedical and legal consequences of your condition and elects to treat you with a blood pressure medicine acceptable to the FAA. The AME knows that it is harder to get you certified if you are on medication.

So the AME coordinates the needed specialists and labs for the reports and tests listed in the cardiovascular protocol. Much time can be saved if the AME collects all the information, puts it into a neat file, and then submits this to the FAA. Forcing the FAA to be the coordinator and facilitator greatly prolongs the process. The data are sent to Oklahoma City to an FAA doctor for the FAA's review and judgment. If a file is complete and straightforward and the AME knows that it will be acceptable, the AME can call the FAA and can often get the authority to certify you over the phone with the condition that the AME will send in the file immediately.

There may be many weeks between the arrival of your application and the evaluation by an FAA doctor. If the file has enough data to justify that the medical condition would not jeopardize your ability to fly safely, the FAA doctor will certify you. In doing this, he or she must consider the data, whether or not your condition is a risk, and how you intend to use your medical certificate. If you are considered not safe to fly, the FAA doctor will send you a letter of denial but will also include instructions on the next step toward reconsideration should you want to take it.

The reason for the denial may be that the FAA doctor does not have the authority to certify you even though the supporting data indicate you could be. You may still have a strong potential for being certified, but you must take your application to the next step: you must request reconsideration *and* special issuance from the Federal Air Surgeon in Washington, D.C. This does not happen automatically; you need to initiate the request.

The information can be reviewed by the Federal Air Surgeon, who has the authority to decide in your favor, ask for more data, or deny you. Yet, even with this denial, the Federal Air Surgeon will suggest a course to follow. The key point is that the Federal Air Surgeon must accept the responsibility of determining whether or not your medical condition is safe for flying. If the problem is more complex than the Federal Air Surgeon wants to judge, a board of specialists will be called upon for further interpretation.

This process of special issuance and reconsideration can also take place at the Oklahoma City level without having to go to the Federal Air Surgeon. In fact, this level has much more authority, and many special issuance files are reviewed here. A panel of specialists will also review more complex files, or a single specialist, not an FAA employee, will be asked to review and recommend what action is appropriate.

In other words, the decision is not an arbitrary one, and every attempt is made to be fair. Remember, determining how your health affects your ability to do any job is like weather forecasting, an inexact science, with data subject to interpretation. Critics of the system may have a valid point, but they are not responsible for ensuring safe flight and do not have to answer to the public.

Although the FAA will make its own conclusion based on the data presented, your doctor's opinion is also considered, especially if he or she is known and respected by the FAA. Often, however, your family doctor, acting in your best interests, may state that there is no reason for you to be grounded when, in fact, he or she is not thoroughly knowledgeable about how your medical condition affects your flying performance. This could mislead you into thinking your problem is less of a danger than it actually is.

Therefore, the doctor you choose to evaluate the data should be knowledgeable about aviation medicine and the certification process. Pilots in a union can get important information and assistance from their aeromedical advisor, a specialist in aviation medicine who is knowledgeable about FAA certification and respected by FAA doctors. Those without a union's help must seek out the necessary assistance from competent aeromedical consultants.

All the data are organized in your file in Oklahoma City or Washington, D.C., for presentation to a contracted specialist or a board. Individual specialists can be used at any time, but the board only meets periodically, approximately every two months. It makes it easier for the FAA to reach a conclusion if all the material is complete and organized when it is sent in. The information is then discussed by the specialist or board of doctors, all specialists in their fields (such as cardiology, internal medicine, or neurology). The specialists are knowledgeable about the effects of your medical condition on flying now and in the future.

The specialist or board of doctors can reach one of the following conclusions:

1. More information is needed, perhaps because it wasn't requested. Thus no decision will be made.

2. You will be certified with some type of monitoring of your medical condition and possibly with a time limit of validity.

3. You will be denied because the data are not adequate to justify certification; had there been a more complete presentation of data, you might have been certified.

4. You will be denied because the FAA believes your medical condition may interfere with your flying now or may lead to an even more hazardous medical problem, and no piece of the substantial data you've supplied the FAA proves otherwise.

It should be obvious that before you present your case to the FAA you should have obtained as much medical data as necessary. Don't second-guess the FAA! Even if your request for reconsideration is denied, you can contact the NTSB (National Transportation Safety Board). However, this is an expensive, prolonged ordeal since you are appealing the legality of the FAA's interpretation of medical regulations.

In other words, because medicine is not an absolute science and there can be several viable and professionally acceptable opinions, the NTSB allows the two sides (your side and that of the FAA) to battle it out in a hearing. Both sides are represented by an attorney. Before taking this action, be sure you have obtained competent medical and legal advice regarding your ability to fly safely with your condition. What you are doing, through an attorney, is claiming that the FAA is wrong in its decision to deny you through its interpretation of the regulations and that you have exhausted all possible avenues for review by the FAA.

For example, say you had a mild stroke, but all the current tests, X rays, angiograms, and other sophisticated data indicate a clean bill of health. The FAA will base its decision on statistical evidence that those who have had a history of stroke have a greater chance of having another, and it will deny you, to be on the safe side. If, on the other hand, you have gathered a commendable collection of data, along with superb legal counsel with expert witnesses, you can challenge this denial to the NTSB (or higher). (However, the NTSB can't change the standards or regulations.) Over the years, the FAA has removed rules and standards that were commonly challenged in court. There are few legal loopholes with which an attorney can plead a case. That may sound like bad news, but keep in mind that medical certification is based on a medical interpretation not a legal one. And, even if you win your medical certification back via the NTSB, be advised that the FAA can appeal the decision and also has the option to keep a close eye on your file.

The FAA provides an appeal process that essentially never ends if you can provide it with additional information that proves you are an acceptable risk for the type of flying you've chosen. With special issuance, history has shown that the Federal Air Surgeon and the FAS office of aviation medicine has certified just about every medical problem there is, except for those that are truly a risk in flight.

A formal denial is required before you can file an appeal with the NTSB. A competent attorney well versed in aviation medicine and law could be a real asset if all else fails. In my opinion, however, this legal route should be used only as a last resort. There are few cases that truly need to be appealed to the NTSB—if you have sought certification properly. If you aren't certified through the customary means, then that usually means that there is still something that the FAA does not approve of, that it does not have enough information, or that not enough time has passed to prove there won't be a progression or recurrence of your disorder.

I am not implying that if you follow these suggestions, you won't have any problems with the FAA. That would be naive and too good to be true. However, the more you can do to better your case and to improve your appeal, the greater chance you will have of a positive result. Certainly you will be way ahead of your colleague with the same medical problem who is waiting for someone else to act.

IN REVIEW

In conclusion, the process of certification may be delayed by two main problems:

1. The inherent bureaucratic sluggishness of review, evaluation, and judgment and of the administrative process of informing you. You have no control over this bureaucratic delay, and you must wait it out like everyone else. Budgetary constraints and reduced staffing make this problem worse.

2. Failure on the part of yourself and your doctors to submit all of the necessary data required by the FAA in one file in an optimal amount of time. This you can control by following my suggestions.

Therefore, in those areas where you can have control, take control. And try not to get too frustrated by those areas that are out of your hands. Better still, avoid this situation in the first place by practicing a good health maintenance program. Here again, there are some critical areas of your health that you can control—and some that you can't. Take control and keep ahead of the FAA. Know what your medical status truly is, and develop a prevention philosophy.

4

Specific Health Problems and Flying

A thirty-eight-year-old airline pilot admits that she is more than usually apprehensive about her FAA exam. She doesn't watch her diet or exercise. When her doctor suggests she change her habits because her blood pressure is creeping up, the combination of all of this is too much. She fails her next FAA exam because her blood pressure is too high. Many months later, in better shape and watching her diet, her blood pressure is controlled but only with medication. She is flying, but every year she has to prove to the FAA that her hypertension is under control.

The following are the most common medical factors that affect a pilot's health and medical certification. (Substance dependence is also a major factor and will be discussed in Chapter 9.) You should become knowledgeable about this information since no pilot is immune to these problems. They include high blood pressure and hypertension, diabetes, coronary artery disease, vision problems, hearing loss, and cardiovascular problems.

HIGH BLOOD PRESSURE AND HYPERTENSION

Elevated blood pressure is one of the more common medical conditions that can ground pilots for weeks or even years. The continual pumping of blood through the blood vessels exerts a certain amount of pressure against the inside walls of the arteries and veins, pushing outward just like the hydraulic system in your aircraft. When the pressure becomes and remains too high, it can damage the arteries, the organs supplied by them, and the pump itself, the heart. Blood pressure is supposed to go up under certain conditions, such as illness, fatigue, too much alcohol or caffeine, and stress. However, it should return to normal when the cause is removed. If it stays elevated, even under normal conditions, this persistent increase in pressure is known as hypertension.

Blood pressure is determined with a tight cuff around the upper arm and a gauge called a "sphygmomanometer" and by using a stethoscope to listen to the sounds of flowing blood in an artery of the arm. The upper number (systolic) is the highest level of pressure within the vessel, and the lower number (diastolic) is the resting pressure before the heart contracts again. Using this method, your doctor can measure your blood pressure at that time. It is not necessarily your true everyday pressure. Many factors influence your blood pressure readings: emotions, fears, environment, position, posture, temperature, time of day, the sight of the medical office and its technicians, and the comments by the doctor, to name a few.

So a diagnosis of hypertension should never be based on only a few readings. Instead, many should be taken over a period of time to find out if the pressure really is up all the time and not just at one particular moment. Sometimes the mere act of repeating blood pressure readings or an idle comment such as "How long has your blood pressure been up?" can keep a professional pilot's blood pressure elevated though it may return to normal as soon as the pilot leaves the doctor's office. Blood pressure from "checkitis" during a simulator check ride is probably the same as from "examitis" or "white coat hypertension"—high!

If your AME takes several blood pressure readings and they all are elevated, this may not necessarily be the result of the hypertension that the FAA is concerned about. High blood pressure from stress is much different than high blood pressure from the disease of hypertension. Also, the FAA will accept a higher blood pressure than your own doctor will accept. Blood pressure in excess of 140/90 is often treated by most doctors with medication, whereas the FAA will accept an untreated blood pressure of 155/95.

Simply establishing the fact that a certain pilot has hypertension or high blood pressure is not the FAA's sole concern. Having high blood pressure may be a manifestation of a disorder that is causing an elevation in pressure. It is that process that must be corrected or reversed, if possible. The cause may be a dietary abuse that can be easily altered, or it may be more serious such as a stricture (sudden narrowing) of an artery or a kidney dysfunction. In any case, it needs to be corrected before any more damage is done by the increased blood pressure. Hypertension is dangerous, even though you may not have any symptoms. The working environment in which you fly—if it leads to sedentary activity, dehydration, hypoxia, or anticipating an emergency—can seriously aggravate even mild hypertension.

There is a misconception that a person with hypertension is hyper or tense. That is not the medical meaning of the word. Also, hypertension is not limited to fat people. Skinny, calm people may also have the same hydraulic pressure problem going on inside their circulatory systems and may need the same treatment. Furthermore, those people may have the false impression that physical appearance and a lack of symptoms are indications of normal blood pressure.

It is common knowledge in the aviation world that many professional pilots consult their family doctors for illness and their AMEs only for their flight physicals. This defeats the real purpose of the flight physical (determining you are fit to fly); it's like cramming for an aviation exam and then disregarding the vitally important information when the exam is over. This practice, although understandable, can be especially threatening to your career because of the usual way that hypertension is treated in most medical communities.

If your personal doctor is not familiar with the FAA's criteria, you could be in for a long ordeal regaining a medical certificate that is denied because of a single elevated blood pressure reading. For example, let's say that your family doctor (not your AME) sees you and says that your blood pressure is "up a bit" or you had a friend take it or you had it taken in a drugstore or at some sports club. The point is if your blood pressure is up it needs to be checked out and, if necessary, treated. Keep in mind that many pilots will see their own doctor for treatment and then see their AME for certification.

Your own doctor may do a few tests to check you out more thoroughly. That's good. I hope your doctor will measure your blood pressure over several days or have you take it at home before tagging you with a diagnosis of hypertension. As I said earlier, in many pilots' cases the mere mention of an elevated blood pressure will be enough to cause an otherwise normal blood pressure to go up as soon as the pilot sees a blood pressure apparatus or a white coat. I hope your private doctor will take this into account before becoming too aggressive in evaluation, diagnosis, and therapy. Too many times I have heard that a pilot was told, "Your blood pressure is too high—you'll probably never fly again." Your blood pressure will never be the same after that remark!

Nevertheless, your doctor can't ignore the fact that your blood pressure is elevated, regardless of the conditions under which it was taken. Recent medical evidence indicates that even mild hypertension (140/90) should be treated, and those with "white coat hypertension" are at greater risk of developing true hypertension in the future. An aggressive doctor could put you on medication for a blood pressure level that is acceptable to the FAA. So what's the best treatment for a pilot? Your doctor can't ignore your high blood pressure because it is dangerous to your health. How can he or she treat your hypertension without grounding you? The answer is that treatment should not be limited to medication.

It is common knowledge that among an inherently healthy population, such as pilots, there is a direct relationship between increased blood pressure and smoking, increased weight, lack of exercise, and consumption of alcohol, caffeine, and too much salt. It is also realized by the medical profession that the odds of the usual patient successfully giving up cigarettes, decreasing alcohol consumption, eliminating unnecessary foods, cutting down on coffee, and beginning a good exercise program are between zero and none. And the typical doctor has little time to try to explain why it is important to avoid these abuses. But the increased blood pressure is still there, so the doctor says, "take this medicine once a day and see me in a couple of weeks," knowing the odds are better that patients will take the pill than change their habits. The doctor may casually add, in passing, "try to lose some weight and get some exercise," but there often is little time spent in explaining how or why.

The blood pressure may be controlled by the medication and you can be certified, but you then have two strikes against you. First, you have a diagnosis of hypertension, and second, you are using medication to control it. Both are disqualifying, at least temporarily, until further evaluated and judged by the FAA. In other words, the FAA rightfully assumes that you have tried all other measures of controlling your blood pressure, such as losing weight, avoiding salt, cutting out cigarettes, and so forth, but to no avail and that medications are the only way your blood pressure (hypertension) can be controlled.

The FAA also reasons that this could mean that you may have severe hypertension (because of your need for medication), and therefore it wants to determine what else could be wrong, such as with your heart, kidneys, or brain. So, the FAA will ask for the "FAA's cardiovascular evaluation," which is very comprehensive and could open the door to more unexplained yet abnormal data—data that now must be reported to the FAA.

The irony is this: your increased blood pressure may not be serious at all and could be controlled simply by avoiding those abuses you should be avoiding anyway, whether you're hypertensive or not. This is another reason for trying to stay ahead of the game by maintaining the good health you brought to the profession.

Having a career or hobby that does not allow you to have significant hypertension or take medication would seem adequate reason for you to follow some commonsense measures of maintaining good physical condition and protecting that valuable career. Yet apathy often causes people to ignore their health until their elevated blood pressure cannot be ignored any longer. Therefore, should your doctor tell you that your blood pressure is up and that you should take medication, ask if you could try some other measures first because medication could jeopardize your career or, at the very least, create a more difficult certification process. These measures include

1. No smoking. I say again, *no* smoking. Fortunately, smoking is not nearly as common among pilots as it was just a few years ago.

2. Reducing your salt intake (salt is sodium chloride). Sodium is the culprit in this case; it's also found in preservatives and in other parts of food, not only in ordinary table salt.

3. Maintaining an ideal weight, a weight your family doctor or your AME should be able to define.

4. Avoiding excessive amounts of caffeine (excessive could range from

one to more than three cups), which is a very strong stimulant and makes the heart work harder than it has to.

5. Avoiding alcohol in more than moderate amounts. The stimulant effects to the heart of excessive alcohol can last for days.

6. Developing an exercise program that is appropriate for you. Initially, it should be under the supervision of a doctor.

As you can see, there is nothing magic about these measures, and nothing that you shouldn't already be doing. By following this very basic program, you greatly reduce the chance of developing an elevated blood pressure as well as many other health problems that would not be acceptable to the FAA, your AME, or your family doctor.

I can't say this enough: waiting for your doctor to tell you that you have something wrong, in this case elevated blood pressure, is not the best way to maintain your health. The odds are great that if you abuse those social amenities in which our society overindulges some disorder will catch up with you. Granted, there is a percentage of pilots who are overweight, smoke, and drink too much and somehow still come through their exams. But the odds for this are small. "Playing the odds" in Las Vegas provides an immediate response. "Playing the odds" with your health will not show results for years. If you want to play those odds, that's up to you; but they're against you! Commonsense measures like watching your diet can improve the odds, and your blood pressure usually can be controlled. Better still, you can keep it from being elevated no matter what the stressful circumstances. By the way, I can abuse my health, take medication, and go back to work. You can't!

Don't assume you can take your health for granted by waiting for hypertension to develop and then working out some way to keep your medical certification. I have worked with too many pilots whose hypertension eventually was easily controlled (by commonsense measures), but the pilot spent many months getting back on the line.

DIABETES

Diabetes is the inability of your body to metabolize or efficiently use essential sugars as fuel. Sugar (to the body) is sugar—no matter what the source. Ultimately, all sugars are metabolized by the body as glucose, which is another common sugar. As a result of this inability to metabolize, the entire body and its organs and tissues are subject to potentially serious complications.

This disorder probably is one of the best-recognized diseases but one of those least understood by the medical profession. It would appear that the more doctors investigate this disease the less they know about it. There is no doubt that diabetes represents a multitude of different problems occurring at the same time within the body—a multiorgan involvement—all of which are deteriorating processes unless brought under control. Therefore, the presence of diabetes severe enough to require medication (that is, not controllable by diet) is a real risk to safe flying. Many dispute the conclusion that diabetes is not safe. They argue that no accidents have been caused by someone with diabetes. What is overlooked is that diabetics, with or without medication, have a higher risk of becoming impaired under the conditions of flight. Even a slight impairment (e.g., mild hypoglycemia, which is common but controllable) can, unpredictably, be enough to distract or incapacitate a pilot during times requiring high concentration and flawless performance. There are obviously exceptions: those whose diabetes is proven to be stable and whom the FAA will consider certifying even if they are on medication.

As far as the FAA is concerned, diabetes is initially ruled out through a urinalysis "dipstick" test during the AME's certification exam. This simply tests your urine for the presence of sugar by a color change on a strip of chemically treated paper. This is, at best, a screening test, and the absence of sugar by that test does not totally rule out the presence of diabetes. But, by the same token, if sugar is present in the urine, then diabetes must be ruled out (for you and the FAA) by additional testing.

There is one disorder called "renal glycosuria," which means that your kidneys spill, or excrete, sugar into the urine under normal circumstances. This is usually an acceptable medical variation once diabetes has been ruled out. The only way to rule out diabetes is to do additional special blood studies, which include a fasting blood sugar (the measurement of sugar in the blood after a minimum of eight hours without any food) and a glucose tolerance test (the hourly measurement of sugar in the blood and the urine following the ingestion of a specified amount of glucose). Both of these tests usually are adequate to identify either the presence or absence of diabetes. Another test, glycosolated hemoglobin (HgbA1c) is also an important part of the evaluation and can tell the doctor how well the body has been responding to glucose metabolism for the previous weeks. However, there are situations where the results are equivocal; that is, the presence or absence of diabetes still cannot be determined absolutely. Therefore, the FAA may require additional evaluations and opinions and often the passage of time to prove stability.

The glucose tolerance test is a controversial evaluation since it has a tendency to overdiagnose. For example, there are some people thought to have diabetes who in fact do not. The diagnosis for these people was based primarily on the glucose tolerance test results, which appeared to be abnormal but were not. In spite of the controversy, the FAA may still require a glucose tolerance test or a two-hour postprandial (testing blood glucose two hours after a meal) to rule out the presence of diabetes if it is suspected. Should you ever be asked to take a glucose tolerance test, be sure that you eat a glucose tolerance test "loading diet" during the three days prior to taking the test. Ask your doctor for the specifics. Keep this in mind: the results of the test are subject to interpretation by a physician, and the same test results could have as many different interpretations as the number of physicians evaluating them.

There are other, more sophisticated blood tests that can be used to more adequately define your "glucose intolerance," and you should check with a specialist to determine which options are in your best interests.

As far as the FAA is concerned, there are upper limits for blood sugar (about 120 for fasting blood sugar and 160 for the two-hour test), but your own doctor may or may not consider those limits acceptable. Diabetics can be certified if their diabetes can be controlled by diet alone, that is, with no use of oral medication or injectable insulin. The FAA quite reasonably assumes that if your diabetes is so severe that it requires medication all other measures, such as diet control, have not worked. It also assumes that there will be other, inevitable complications that are common with any diabetic (cardiovascular problems being the most significant).

Therefore, should there be any suspicion that you have diabetes, it behooves you to make the utmost effort to follow a strict diabetic diet and structured exercise program (now recognized as a key to non–insulin-dependent diabetes control) to give yourself every possible chance to control it without medication. Once your doctor decides that you must remain on medication, especially injectable insulin, that could be the end of your flying career until you can prove that you have control of the diabetes. Some oral hypoglycemics are approved for use in controlling diabetes, but a more thorough evaluation and risk assessment is expected by the FAA.

I have seen several cases where sugar has appeared for the first time in the urine of a pilot who has an extra amount of fat, overindulges in pastries, enjoys more than an occasional beer, and is generally out of shape. Almost invariably, with better control of dietary intake of carbohydrates, loss of weight, and exercise, this tendency to spill sugar can be reduced, and no further action is necessary. In other words, the presence of sugar in the urine can be a result of poor diet. However, until proven otherwise, sugar's presence has to be assumed as indicating early diabetes.

CORONARY ARTERY DISEASE

Coronary artery disease (CAD) is one of the significant causes of both permanent and temporary medical certificate denials. The current FAR Part 67 states that even a history of coronary artery disease requires mandatory certificate denial by your Aviation Medical Examiner until you can prove the disease is stable and does not generate any impairment during flight and at altitude. There is good reason for this rule since anyone with coronary artery disease does have a greater risk of developing a heart attack or other disabling conditions leading to sudden incapacitation. Once coronary artery disease is detected through any means, it cannot be ignored—CAD is a progressive disease. Recent studies show, however, that the process can be reversed with a good health and cardiac maintenance program. These rules put professional pilots in a quandary. If they have no CAD symptoms, should they avoid looking for something that may ground them? Or should they look for something with the idea that if a problem does turn up they will correct it to save their lives and to protect their medical certificates?

Coronary arteries are the vessels that bring necessary blood to the heart muscle. Heart muscle is like any other muscle in the body and requires oxygen and nutrients to function. The heart is simply a pump in the body's hydraulic system—and you only have one pump. This hydraulic system is a closed system in which arteries take oxygen and nutrient-rich blood to all parts of the body and blood is brought back to the heart via the veins. Coronary artery disease is either a plugging up of coronary arteries or a stiffening or thickening of the walls of the arteries, greatly compromising the ability of the arteries to bring blood to the heart muscle. If there is too little blood and therefore inadequate oxygen and nutrients, either chest pain (angina pectoris) develops or a myocardial infarction (a heart attack, a condition where blood is completely cut off) occurs. When blood supply from an artery is compromised (reduced), that is called "ischemia." Unfortunately, ischemia doesn't always result in symptoms or angina. If one has ischemia, it is unpredictable as to how that will progress to a complete blockage.

Most medical professionals generally agree that coronary artery disease is a result of an abnormal amount of cholesterol either within the wall of the artery or as formations of plaque or obstructions along the inside of the walls of the artery. Whether or not this cholesterol in the coronary arteries is directly related to the amount of cholesterol in your blood is a subject of much disagreement, but there is a direct relationship between the amount of cholesterol in your blood and the *risk* of developing coronary artery disease, and therefore it is an important risk factor. Thus, knowing cholesterol levels, along with other test results (HDL, the "good cholesterol"; triglycerides; and LDL), is a very important part of determining your odds of developing coronary artery disease in the future.

Many good books and frequent articles refer to the relationship of cholesterol and other factors to the development of coronary artery disease. My purpose is not to duplicate these efforts but to state basic facts and to let you come to your own conclusions.

Recognized independent risk factors, that is, those abuses that by themselves greatly increase the odds of professional pilots developing coronary artery disease and losing their careers, are age, increased blood pressure (or hypertension), cigarette smoking, family history of coronary artery disease, sedentary lifestyle, high cholesterol, diabetes, and being male. Only three of these variables are beyond your control—heritage of a family history of coronary artery disease, age, and gender. The variables you can control are obvious and well recognized by everyone even minimally versed in good health maintenance.

Consider this: if the treatment for high blood pressure or coronary artery disease is diet control, the development of a good exercise program, and the avoidance of cigarettes, alcohol, excessive caffeine, and high-fat foods, why not begin such therapy before developing the disease that could take away your certificate? This does require effort, but unfortunately you picked a career that requires you to maintain your health. I don't think you need the threat of the bureaucratic FAA taking away your certificate to force you into following a good, commonsense health maintenance program. Crisis management is not a good practice.

Anyone with severe coronary artery disease cannot safely fly an airplane. This is because, at altitude, oxygen partial pressure is reduced, adding even more stress to the heart muscle than already is present because of the CAD, and the potential for heart failure is increased. This can lead to sudden death, incapacitation, or a subtle impairment of performance. However, flying with CAD is a controversial subject since there are prominent physicians who say that there is no added risk to flying and the pilot will know when not to fly if there is heart disease present. Few aeromedical doctors agree with this. In any case, if you can control risk factors that are likely to lead to CAD and likely to end your career, it would seem prudent to begin to work on some sort of health maintenance program now.

It is very common to see pilots develop hypertension or CAD solely as a result of allowing their physical condition to deteriorate. Some studies say that if we did angiograms (X rays of the coronary arteries) on the U.S. population, a significant percentage already would have CAD without symptoms. Many times this unsuspected CAD is found indirectly as a result of testing for an unrelated problem, such as high blood pressure. High blood pressure may require exercise cardiac stress testing for certification by the FAA, and the stress test is often the first indication that CAD is present. I am not advocating ignoring a medical problem, but if a doctor is forced to look for one, chances are he or she will find something wrong and will have to report this to the FAA, and your career is on the line.

Therefore, if you can avoid hypertension by following a health maintenance program, additional tests (that could lead to discovery of other problems not medically significant) will not be necessary. I refer you to the last section of this chapter on cardiac stress testing to illustrate how many pilots are grounded for unsuspected disorders when, had they just followed some health maintenance program, they could have avoided this.

Bypass surgery, a medically common procedure for correcting (but not curing) CAD, is a subject of concern to professional pilots. It is difficult, but not uncommon, for pilots who have had a heart attack or significant CAD to regain medical certificates allowing them to fly in any seat of responsibility, especially in the left seat of an airliner. Bypass surgery, which involves by-passing the clogged coronary artery with another implanted vessel (actually a leg vein), does, in fact, improve blood flow to that part of the heart muscle. However, it does not remove the initial cause of the progressive CAD; it does not cure heart disease.

Other procedures for treatment include angioplasty and stents. Your health is primary, but if there is a choice of procedures, check with your AME as to which ones are the most and least acceptable to the FAA.

While these surgeries will not cure CAD, they will improve your health. Only time will tell whether or not they remove the future risk of incapacita-tion. Therefore, the FAA will reconsider someone who has had bypass surgery, depending upon the results, how much time has passed, and whether or not the pilot has been able to control other risk factors. If ischemia is found in any test, the pilot will usually not be certified. This is a situation that can be reversed through proper health maintenance. Keep in mind, however, that this individ-ual has a history of significant CAD and still has the disease and therefore will face a mandatory denial by an AME until further evaluation.

A key point bears repeating. CAD is a common problem, and it alone can ground you, either temporarily or permanently. Don't wait to be told you have CAD before you control your controllable risk factors.

VISION PROBLEMS

Testing your visual acuity, that is, your ability to see near or distant objects (with or without glasses), obviously is an important part of determining your ability to fly safely. Most of you have had enough vision tests to know what the procedure is. However, there are occasions where the instrument (other than an eye chart) used for determining visual acuity could distort results because this instrument uses a series of mirrors to simulate distance. Therefore, if you have borderline results, make sure that you have your vision checked either with an eye chart in a well-lit eye lane or by being examined by an ophthal-mologist or optometrist.

Most abnormal distant vision changes occur before age twenty-two, and your vision might even improve during the next few years that follow. But after that, your vision will remain relatively stable, especially your distant vision. As you pass forty, your near vision will begin to deteriorate, and reading glasses will be necessary. Your first indication that there may be a change is during night flying—the charts will be harder to read.

Abnormal near vision is corrected for reading to allow you to focus on a book or newspaper without too much difficulty. Keep in mind that as a pilot much of your near vision work is done at the instrument panel, the console or pedestal, and where you normally look at your approach plates. This location could be several feet farther than the distance at which you hold books. Everyone's near vision will deteriorate with age, usually after age forty. This is called "presbyopia" and is a predictable change. Many older pilots will not wear their reading glasses until they realize during a flight that they can't read the charts or the instruments, usually at night.

Reading glasses are essential if your uncorrected near visual acuity is less than 20/20. Primarily when you are fatigued and hypoxic and in low light (e.g., just before a descent after a long trip at night), your near vision will be impaired. Consequently, you should let your eye doctor know that you are a pilot so that glasses can be prescribed that give you sharp 20/20 vision, both distant and near. The revised vision testing now includes intermediate near vision after age fifty. So, distances of 16 and 32 inches will be checked. Remember, testing for vision in the doctor's office is done when you are rested and not hypoxic and are in a well-lit room. Bifocals may be necessary to improve your vision, and you may need trifocals to see the instrument panels clearly. Bifocals are also available where the correction is at the top of the lens for looking up at the overhead panel.

Glasses and conventional contact lenses are accepted by the FAA as long as they adequately correct your visual deficiency. The most thorough exam is to test for your refractive error. This is a technique by which the eye doctor can determine the actual ability of your eye to focus without correction. In most cases, the FAA will certify pilots with bad uncorrected vision as long as their corrected vision is 20/20 in *both* eyes. It is always a good idea to have your vision checked by an eye doctor periodically in addition to the FAA exam.

Contact lenses are also acceptable: they do not require any waiver for use and are sometimes better than frame glasses because they improve peripheral vision. Be sure that you follow the instructions for the type of contacts you use. Extended wear contacts are not recommended.

A lot is said about using Ortho K (orthokeratology) to correct vision so that lenses don't have to be worn for hours or even days. In this technique, a special kind of hard contact lens physically molds the cornea of the eye. The result in some is improved visual acuity for a short period of time when the contact lens is removed. Obviously, this is a popular technique for young pilots wanting to be hired by a company that accepts pilots with uncorrected 20/20 vision only. However, this is no longer an issue since there is no longer an uncorrected standard and a company cannot inquire about an applicant's medical status prior to issuing a job offer (a result of the Americans with Disability Act [ADA]). Furthermore, this correction is temporary, at best, and it is still a correction. And what happens if you lose a contact or get a corneal scratch, common with hard contacts, and you can't wear your contacts for a day or so? You must wear frame glasses again. The FAA accepts Ortho K, but the pilot still is responsible for seeing 20/20 while in flight.

Another technique, radial keratotomy, is a form of refractive surgery whereby slits cut in the front of the cornea resemble the spokes of a wheel. As these cuts heal, they change the contour of the cornea, and vision can be corrected. Other similar techniques use lasers "to carve" the cornea. The down side is that there are still unpredictable problems in up to 20 percent of the cases and it's expensive. My feeling is that you shouldn't have surgery on a perfectly normal eye that can be corrected with lenses. Why take any risk if your medical certificate could be in jeopardy? The same is true for the new laser correction. It's still surgery.

Testing for glaucoma is no longer expected for FAA medical certification. However, a field of vision test is, and that will be abnormal if the glaucoma is advanced. If you have a family history of glaucoma, you should have it checked. Otherwise, after age thirty-five, it should be a part of your vision exam by the eye doctor. Glaucoma is increased pressure within the eyeball. As pressure increases in the eye, it will gradually destroy the retina and the ability to see. This is a permanent change leading to progressive blindness. If you wait until you begin to notice changes in your vision, rather than being regularly tested for glaucoma, damage may have already been done. Glaucoma that has been brought under control with eyedrops before the vision has deteriorated is certifiable by the FAA.

Color blindness is not really an acceptable term any more. We now know that there are variations in color vision, so a better term is *color deficiency*. It is usually a permanent, unchanging condition. However, it may change as you get older and the lens or cornea becomes discolored from the aging process; this can be the first sign of a cataract. The main purpose of the color vision test is to determine if you, as a pilot, are able to detect red and green, especially at night. Are the red and green lights in front of you approaching or departing? The runway approach lights are often red and green (e.g., VASI is red). With the high-tech cockpit using more colors to determine aircraft performance, normal color vision becomes more essential. Therefore, the screening test usually used in a doctor's office is to determine the presence of color deficiency severe enough to compromise safety. If you miss a certain number of plates in the test, you are considered color deficient. Some people cannot make out the characters because of the type of light in the exam room. If you are having trouble, ask to have the test done in actual sunlight. Unless you can clearly make out colors, the instrument panel with all its colors and hues might be difficult to read. (Is that character an *8,* a *3,* a *B,* or a *0?*)

A more accurate test, the color threshold test, uses different-colored lights at varying intensities; it may show that you are color deficient yet color safe.

This test, done only in the military, is unfortunately no longer made. However, the FAA will accept its results if you can access the test. Another test, the Farnsworth lantern test (FALANT), is also acceptable to the FAA, but once again it is normally found only in the military. However, some eye doctors will have the FALANT or other acceptable color vision tests, so checking around to see who has the test may be worth your time if you know you are color deficient.

The 1996 amended standards simply state, "Ability to perceive colors necessary for the safe performance of airman duties." The *Guide for Aviation Medical Examiners* further defines what is expected depending on the class requested and the pilot's duties. For a second- or third-class medical certificate, the FAA will allow a waiver if you can pass a light gun test. This test uses a light gun (as is used in an ATC tower) to determine whether or not you can distinguish between red and green. However, for a first-class medical certificate, a more critical evaluation is required. A medical flight test (check ride) must be completed. The examiner will fly with you (or taxi around the field) in various conditions during the day and night, making sure that you can distinguish the VASI, radio towers, approaching traffic, and taxiways, among other things. If you can, there is no problem with the certification, and you will be given a Statement of Demonstrated Ability (SODA). If you can't, then obviously you shouldn't be flying at night, especially in high-traffic areas. All these additional tests must be authorized by the FAA doctors at Oklahoma City before you take them. Your AME can assist in this coordination by requesting the FAA to authorize you to take one of these tests.

Depth perception testing was once considered to be an important part of your visual evaluation. Today there is no requirement for this test. Depth perception (having both of your eyes working together to determine the distance of objects) is only critical up to about twenty feet. Beyond that, depth perception is based on visual cues. That is, over the years, your eyes and your brain have become familiar with the relative sizes of different objects; for example, if you see a distant tree with a car next to it, you know the approximate size of each and are able to judge how far you are from them. This is why the 747 looks so slow while it is flying. Your brain's "computer" is not used to that large an aircraft, and it appears to be closer and thus slower than it really is. However, if you flew a 727 at the same speed right underneath a 747, the relative size of the 747 would be most apparent, as well as its speed.

Along with this, different visual cues used to perceive an object on a clear day may be masked by haze or fog. The main point is that depth perception testing is not as critical as one would expect, unless there is marked inability to fuse the eyes to see objects less than twenty feet away. This is what is called "bifoveal fixation," where both eyes are focusing on the same object. It is easily evaluated at the time of the physical exam and can be corrected by glasses.

Being unable to fuse both eyes on the same object is called a "phoria" or "tropia," and this is tested during the eye exam. If you have an extreme case of phoria, double vision can occur, especially when you are tired or hypoxic.

Space myopia occurs while you are flying at altitude on a clear day. In other words, you have nothing distant to focus on, such as a cloud, when you look out the window. If you find yourself staring out the window, move your eyes around more: look around the cockpit occasionally and look back at the wingtip. By not focusing on something distant, you may not be able to see a distant object clearly if it does appear, such as traffic not pointed out by ATC.

All of these situations can be minimized if your vision is corrected and you know your deficiencies. Avoiding the wearing of glasses does no good, despite what you may hear (such as "not wearing glasses strengthens the eyes"). In fact not wearing glasses will cause eye strain. Wear glasses if you need them.

HEARING LOSS

The ability to hear is almost as important as the ability to see. Although some of today's flying is done with computers and visual displays, your hearing still cannot be replaced for coordinating your flight with that of others in your airspace or detecting sounds that are related to the performance of the aircraft. Unlike poor vision, poor hearing cannot be corrected. A hearing aid or wearing a headset is acceptable for some kinds of hearing loss in flight. But this is a distraction, and the loss might have been preventable. Therefore, the preservation of your hearing is most important.

For professional pilots to communicate, only the voice range is important: 500 to 2,000 cycles per second (Hz). Your airplane's communication system is not high fidelity. That is, it is not burdened with having to communicate the higher and lower frequencies beyond the voice range. That is why the FAA's evaluation of hearing only includes voice range. As far as the FAA is concerned, if you have acceptable hearing of voice frequencies, it does not matter if you can't hear the other ones. And often people do develop high-frequency hearing loss.

The only true way to evaluate your hearing is with the audiometer, the results of which are recorded as a hearing curve called the "audiogram." The old whispered voice test is archaic and gives no objective, quantitative data. The current "voice" test is better but still doesn't quantify hearing loss. Audiometry must be performed in a quiet room with an adequate, well-calibrated instrument. The audiometry test done in most doctors' offices are screening tests at best, and if you suspect any hearing loss, you should have your hearing checked by an audiologist, someone who specializes in the determination of hearing ability. Even a screening test is better than a simple conversation test.

Although the FAA is interested only in your ability to hear frequencies in the voice range, you and your AME should also be interested in the higher frequencies. If a high-frequency hearing loss is detected, it is an indication that you are probably being subjected to excessive noise, because high-frequency hearing loss is most often the result of exposure to noise. This is an indication of a progressive deterioration. It is said that flight surgeons could often determine the type of airplanes (fighters and bombers) World War II aviators flew and their crew positions based on the degree of their high-frequency hearing loss and which ear was affected. In today's aviation, many cockpits are still noisy, and ramps are worse. And you are always exposed to noise if you use a chain saw, lawn mower, or home woodworking equipment. If you're losing high-frequency hearing through exposure to noise, this exposure may ultimately affect your ability to hear frequencies in the voice range, and a waiver or SODA will be required. The only way that you can detect this deterioration is through a well-performed audiometry test.

Hearing loss from noise, which probably accounts for the greatest percentage of hearing loss in the pilot, can be prevented easily by the unsophisticated methods of using ear plugs and noise-attenuating headsets. Since a change may be insidious, wear protection in noisy areas.

How do you tell if you are in an area noisy enough to produce hearing loss? An area that will subject you to some hearing loss probably is best described as any area in which you must raise your voice above a normal speaking level for any length of time or if your normal voice can't be heard from about three feet away. Don't forget to use protection even in your home activities. There is a product called Ears, a sponge rubber–type ear plug, which I have found to be most effective and comfortable. A pair is inexpensive and easily carried in a flight bag. By the way, prolonged exposure to noise is also very fatiguing.

When doing physical exams on pilots, I often ask them if they have ever had an ear block. There is either a passive no or an emphatic yes! Those who have had an ear block never want another one. Ear blocks occur quite commonly when flying with a cold or allergies. An ear block results from the inability of the eustachian tube to equalize pressure on both sides of the eardrum. As the aircraft and cabin altitude climb, the pressure decreases within the middle ear.

With an ear block, air going out of the middle ear quite easily escapes through the congested eustachian tube. However, on descent, the air cannot get back through the congested eustachian tube, and a negative pressure results within the middle ear. The external increase in pressure on the eardrum now begins to push it inward, creating severe pain plus an additional ear block as a result of the swelling created by the block itself. If you are caught in this situation, you should relieve the block immediately, if at all possible, by returning to an altitude above that at which the ear block began. That is, raise the cabin altitude beyond where you were level and then slowly decrease it. The Valsalva maneuver will also assist: hold your nose and then blow against that resistance. There are other techniques that people use, such as cracking their jaws, swallowing, and shaking their heads. The important point is that the pressure must be equalized before reaching ground. Otherwise, severe damage can result. If you take a chance and fly with a cold, you may develop an ear block that requires weeks to resolve. You will also be temporarily grounded. Some of the oral decongestants that can be bought over the counter, such as Sudafed, are quite effective for mild congestion.

The important thing to remember is to begin to clear your ears as soon as a block develops. Don't wait for it to become worse before doing a Valsalva. Also, a long-acting nose spray, such as Afrin, is good to keep in your flight bag if you get caught in flight with a block. Overuse of any over-the-counter nose sprays will result in a rebound effect, causing congestion. Be sure the decongestant has no antihistamines because they can cause drowsiness. Read the label. As with any self-medication, if you have symptoms significant enough to warrant medication, you probably shouldn't be flying.

A sinus block is similar to an ear block except that the sinuses are involved. The sinuses are located over the forehead and on both sides of the nose around the cheek bone. Again, anyone who has had a sinus block does not want a repeat performance. The techniques used for relieving ear blocks are used for sinus blocks except for the Valsalva, which is not very effective.

Ear wax can also impede hearing. Some people feel that it is absolutely mandatory that all traces of ear wax be removed and will use all sorts of techniques to get it out, everything from toothpicks and hairpins to flushing with water. However, grandma's old rule of "Stick nothing smaller than your elbow into in your ear" is still relevant. Unless the wax is obstructing the entire lumen of the ear canal, the wax is actually there for a purpose. It prevents foreign bodies, such as dust and bugs, from entering. However, after swimming or taking a shower, you might find that your ear wax forms a dam and holds water behind it, which will cause a decrease in hearing until cleared.

THE FAA'S CARDIOVASCULAR EVALUATION AND CARDIAC STRESS TESTING

If your AME and/or the FAA determine during your routine FAA exam that you may have a cardiovascular problem (e.g., elevated blood pressure or an abnormal ECG), the FAA will require additional medical data before it will certify you. This more thorough physical is outlined in the FAA's protocol for a cardiovascular evaluation (see page 58). It is not routinely done unless there is a suspected problem.

This FAA cardiovascular evaluation is like any other comprehensive medical evaluation by your own doctor. A complete physical usually includes a thorough history and a physical examination. In addition, a chest X ray and battery of blood tests and resting ECG test are common. This kind of evaluation is essential in any good health maintenance program and is required by the FAA. Based upon these data, the doctor usually is able to make a fairly valid interpretation of your overall health. With that as a basis, your doctor might add more elaborate tests to evaluate any suspected medical disorders more completely.

However, an additional test in the FAA's cardiovascular evaluation is sometimes required—the cardiac exercise ECG test, or a stress test. The stress test, although a very valuable medical tool, is subject to considerable controversy depending upon whom you are talking with and within what medical community you have the test.

At this point I would like to make it perfectly clear that the opinions expressed here are my own. In addition, I am in no way advocating that a potential or suspected cardiovascular disorder be ignored. However, each time physicians evaluate patients, they consider the effectiveness, the necessity, the risk factors, and the economics involved, along with the element of time, before subjecting the patients to these sophisticated tests solely to determine a diagnosis. It is common knowledge that there are many medical tests available that can tell us a lot, but some are extremely expensive and complex and therefore are not done routinely. Some of these tests add a risk factor and are reserved for special medical problems.

Using this philosophy to determine the necessity of any test for an individual, you must consider that in a professional pilot's situation a cardiac stress test is potentially threatening. Part of a doctor's Hippocratic oath is to do no harm. A stress test might ruin a pilot's career. Therefore, a doctor who considers a stress test must weigh its effect on a pilot's career against its need in the diagnostic process. The reasoning for this is simple: *an abnormal (or positive) stress test is an indication of a heart disorder until proven otherwise.* Yet it is a medically accepted fact that up to 20 percent or more of patients with abnormal results from cardiac stress tests are actually found to be free of any abnormality after subsequent and more sophisticated tests are done. Most people—those who don't fly for a living—return to work during these subsequent tests. A pilot, however, can be grounded until the suspected disorder is ruled out. Also, in up to 20 percent of the tests, someone with a negative result actually has CAD.

Keeping this in mind, let us discuss the cardiac stress test and its implication on a pilot's career. Stress tests basically are performed for three reasons: (1) your doctor suspects that you have a diseased heart or a potential problem with your cardiovascular system, (2) you begin an exercise program, or (3) they are needed for screening purposes in preventive medicine or a prehiring/placement exam. It is important that the techniques used to perform stress tests be the same so that all results have a comparable meaning.

Basically you are connected by a series of wires to an ECG machine so you can be monitored at all times with a continuous tracing during exercise. Then the doctor increases the resistance on the bicycle or raises the incline of the treadmill so you must work harder, which consequently increases your pulse rate. The doctor, before the test, will have determined a target rate based mainly upon your age.

As you work harder, the heart's pumping rate increases. As this happens, the doctor monitors the ECG, looking for abnormalities such as a change in the regularity of your heart beat, blood pressure, and other symptoms. The doctor is not only looking for how long or fast you can run, although that is important. (The stress test should be done in facilities capable of taking care of cardiovascular emergencies. People with unsuspected heart problems have had cardiac arrests or equally serious problems during the test.)

The doctor is looking for indications of irregularities on the ECG that suggest a current or old heart attack (or myocardial infarction), ischemia (reduced blood supply), blocks to the electrical conduction of current that is essential in a functioning heart, and other abnormalities. As mentioned, a medical problem is considered abnormal until proven otherwise, depending upon why you are being examined, what sort of symptoms you have, and the status of your complete physical condition. The doctor may elect to do additional tests because the findings, although valuable, are not sensitive or complete enough to finalize a diagnosis. The doctor may repeat the test, get a second opinion, and, after equivocal findings, may subject you to more sophisticated and expensive tests such as a thallium scan or the ultimate test, the coronary angiogram (or catheterization).

Of course, the perfect evaluation would be obtained by opening you up and looking at the coronary arteries as is done during an autopsy. These arteries bring blood and oxygen to the heart muscle. We are concerned about any one or all of these arteries in a cardiovascular evaluation. All the tests—except physically looking at the arteries and the coronary angiogram—are implicit tests. This means we infer the condition of the coronary arteries by the tests we have done.

Stress tests are simple screening tests in most cases, and many doctors do not feel a stress test is appropriate during a routine exam unless there are clinical reasons for it or the patient is at risk of having heart disease. A stress test is not as effective in determining the condition of the arteries as the thallium scan, the echo stress ECG test, and the angiogram. Currently, the angiogram is the only test that can determine the true status of your coronary arteries, the only test that proves to the FAA that your coronary arteries are not significantly diseased. If you have an abnormal stress test, you may be grounded until it's proven that the results are not disqualifying for flying duties or that you are an acceptable risk in flight despite the medical findings. It often is difficult to determine just how much of a risk your condition is, partly because of the disease's unpredictability of progression and how it could impair a pilot during flight.

Knowing this, why would a pilot undergo a stress test? Well, first of all, most pilots are interested in their health, and therefore some will occasionally get into an exercise program like those at the YMCA, athletic clubs, or schools. Managers of conditioning programs suggest that you have a stress test before beginning so that you can determine the physical condition of your heart and protect yourself and them from an unsuspected heart problem. Usually this means that your own doctor should certify that there is no reason you couldn't follow the conditioning program. The stress test usually is an appropriate way for your doctor to make such a recommendation.

Another reason for the stress test is the preplacement or company periodic physical exam. Again, this would detect unsuspected heart disease that could show up at a later date. A resting ECG would not rule out many such problems.

Yet another reason for the stress test is the FAA or company cardiovascular evaluation. As you know, a resting ECG is required by the FAA at age thirty-five and then annually after age forty for a first-class certificate. If you have an abnormal ECG or a change in your resting ECG, the FAA may want the cardiovascular evaluation done.

There is no big deal about taking a cardiac stress test, except for that clinker—the false positives. Therefore, all this evaluation could come about not because of heart disease but because a medical problem that could have been prevented was not.

As I mentioned before, I am not advocating ignoring a medical disorder. If you are a responsible pilot, you are not ignoring their health, and as a part of your job you have periodic examinations. And if you follow a good health maintenance program, you don't need a stress test to confirm your heart condition. If you can keep a step ahead of the situation, then the chance of your having an unsuspected heart problem is very small. If handled properly, there should be no threat in the stress test. However, if you have allowed yourself to be in a situation where a stress test is required and that stress test happens to be a false positive, there is only one person to blame for being grounded, especially if that test proves something you have always suspected—that you are out of shape.

So what do you do? A stress test can be a valid test, but it can have a direct bearing on your flying career. If it is required by the FAA, there is nothing that you can do. Just keep your fingers crossed and hope that everything works out. Be sure, however, that it is monitored by a knowledgeable AME who is familiar with the FAA's criteria and the interpretation of the stress test. But as I mentioned before, don't wait for this evaluation to be thrown at you as a result of your poor physical conditioning or poor control of risk factors.

If you intend to begin an exercise program, which I advocate, the necessity of a stress test should be determined by your doctor, who should know about the FAA criteria. Your doctor may feel that, all things considered, the stress test is not needed. However, in view of your physical and medical condition and your age and the type of program you are starting, the doctor may require the stress test. If this is the case, then I would certainly agree with this necessity, especially if the doctor suspects a cardiovascular disease.

Most importantly, remember what could develop from a test that need not have been done. So let me repeat these key points regarding the stress test: It is a valid tool and definitely has its place, but its interpretation may be subjective and can result in false positives. You can avoid an unnecessary stress test, which must be reported to the FAA. Be sure that your doctor is informed about the criteria you must meet and the impact that a false positive will have on your career. An abnormal stress test result cannot be ignored since it is an indication of a cardiac disorder until proven otherwise with additional tests and it could lead to unnecessary grounding.

The cardiovascular evaluation provides useful information. It is essential for evaluating your true status and either confirming your good health or detecting a potential progressive disorder that may, if untreated, lead to being grounded prematurely. It's an important evaluation, but wouldn't it be better not to have to report it to the FAA?

NOTE: There are other disorders that can interfere with flying, some which need an AME's OK as well as the FAA's. These disorders include a kidney stone, an ulcer, migraine headaches, fainting for an unknown reason, and other unpredictable conditions. Those who have had one of these medical problems are at higher risk of a recurrence than those who have not. Consequently, your AME needs to know when you have an ulcer or a kidney stone. Technically, flying with a disorder violates FAR 61.53 because it is a deficiency that could recur in flight. Take a look at the items listed in item 18 of Application Form 8500-8. Just about everything that is listed there should be reviewed by your AME before flying.

IN REVIEW

The FAA expects pilots to be free of any medical problem that would interfere with safe flight, a problem that could lead to impairment or even a subtle incapacitation. This obviously is the reason for periodic medical examinations by a physician familiar with flight physiology. Symptoms are not the sole indication of fitness for flight—feeling good doesn't mean you are free of a medical disorder.

The more common ailments of concern in aviation are cardiovascular and neurological system disorders, diabetes, and vision and hearing problems. It is important that you recognize that if you are suspected of having these problems you must be evaluated to prove to yourself and the FAA that you are fit to fly. Keeping ahead of the FAA by participating in a health maintenance program is even smarter. Be sure, however, that someone familiar with aviation, flight physiology, and FAA medical standards reviews any test findings with you. And you must be familiar with the options available for evaluating your health and correcting medical problems.

With this insight, you can be more confident when taking your FAA exam, and you will have a better idea of what to expect from your AME. Waiting until a doctor finds something that doesn't meet FAA standards is a true case of crisis management. I've given you the insight; now it's up to you to follow through.

5

How to Work with Your Family Doctor and AME

A thirty-three-year-old pilot had some mild chest pain on his left side. His resting ECG was slightly abnormal. His cardiac stress test was also slightly abnormal. Although he was not an AME, the doctor, who was terrified of flying, told the pilot that, although he had not had a heart attack, he had a heart problem and would never fly again. The pilot, believing this, and being completely discouraged, grounded himself and did not seek guidance from an aeromedical doctor for several months. Once he did, however, further studies and interpretation by an aviation-oriented physician convinced the FAA that the pilot did not have a disqualifying or unsafe disorder.

We come now to the second part of the book. You now know why you must be healthy, how your health affects your flying performance and being a safe pilot, and how the FAA certifies your good health. Now you need to put that knowledge to work.

An obvious reason for professional pilots having a health maintenance program is to increase longevity so that they can keep flying until retirement and continue flying for fun afterward. Staying healthy until their sixtieth year plus one day may be a secondary challenge, but being able to remain productive at any age is more important. Continued good health is the key to a productive, rewarding, fulfilling life, and keeping this in proper perspective, with realistic priorities, is a challenge. One might think that pilots, getting frequent medical exams throughout their careers, would not have to be concerned about following a health maintenance program. But they should be even though they often perceive more extensive medical evaluation as a potential threat.

THE COMPLACENCY OF HEALTH MAINTENANCE

It is relatively common for professional pilots to seek medical care or a medical interpretation of their health from a family doctor and then to seek FAA medical certification from another, nonthreatening, FAA examiner. (In other words, "If I feel OK, why look for trouble?") Pilots do this because they are afraid they will lose their medical certification and career—no small matter.

This behavior could, however, be the source of problems for the pilot who unknowingly has a medical problem. Your family doctor has a responsibility to you and so does the FAA examiner. However, as discussed earlier, your family doctor usually is not aware of your unique aeromedical requirements, the FAA requirements and expectations, and the effect of the medical disorder and its treatment on your safe flying performance. In contrast, your FAA medical examiner probably doesn't know much about you since you have been reluctant to admit anything more than you absolutely have to in order to pass your FAA physical.

Let me use an example of hypertension (persistent high blood pressure) to explain this "triple-standard dilemma"—your standard for health, your doctor's, and the FAA's. I use hypertension as an example since it is very common and involves a medical disorder with which we are all familiar, one that often leads to a pilot being grounded or having certification delayed. The sequence of events is the same for any medical problem known or suspected.

If you have been diagnosed as having hypertension, your family doctor will probably treat you immediately with medication. Why? A religiously followed health maintenance program that includes, for example, weight loss, exercise, avoidance of salts, and no smoking may lower your blood pressure. However, your doctor knows from experience that most patients won't comply with this program, but he or she has little time for the futility of explaining this. The hypertension can't be ignored, so your doctor puts you on medication because it will lower your blood pressure and because you will take it more readily than you will follow a health maintenance program. This is an appropriate way to treat hypertension.

But this medication, along with the presence of high blood pressure, disqualifies your medical certification until you are more completely evaluated. Before prescribing medication, a competent AME who notices that your blood pressure is elevated and that you are out of shape and overweight will suggest lowering your blood pressure through a health maintenance program.

THE ROLE OF YOUR DOCTOR(S)

Since you do not commonly consult your AME if you have an illness, let's discuss how you can work with your family doctor in preparation for your exam by the FAA no matter what disorder you have. We will first discuss how a physician in private practice, that is, your family doctor, usually functions. Your family doctor's primary purpose and concern is to protect your health and treat anything that interferes with maintaining it. He or she will also advise you on good health maintenance practices. Secondarily, your doctor is just as anxious to get you back to work as you are. Quite frequently, when a doctor feels that a patient can work, he or she will tell that patient's company that its employee can return to work with or without any restrictions. That note from the doctor is usually adequate justification to the company to allow the employee to return to work. The doctor has the credentials and the authority to do this. This is not true for pilots. Just because your doctor says you can return to work without restrictions, that does not mean that you have met the requirements of the FAA. There is a great difference in having a medical disorder that is treatable to your doctor's satisfaction and a medical disorder that is certifiable to the FAA's satisfaction. That is, many disorders that are controlled may not necessarily be aeromedically safe for flying until proven to be safe. Your disorder has to be considered unacceptable until proven otherwise.

The practice of medicine is similar to meteorology. It is not an exact science, and interpretations of medical data vary. To evaluate and treat you, your doctor will use his or her training and expertise and experience with other patients with similar symptoms. You usually see your family doctor only when you have some symptoms that you cannot explain. Your doctor's first objective is to review the symptoms that you report (such as an ache, swelling, or fever) to diagnose the cause. Then, based upon that diagnosis, he or she will treat you with appropriate medication or other therapy.

MAKING THE DIAGNOSIS, NOT JUST TREATING SYMPTOMS

Depending upon the severity of the suspected illness, a doctor may use as many tests as necessary to evaluate a problem. If the doctor still can't explain symptoms that could indicate a more serious disorder, he or she will do even more tests and probably consult with other doctors to come to a responsible conclusion. Remember, the doctor is seeing you because you are coming in with symptoms, which must be related to a cause. Doctors do not treat symptoms as much as the cause of those symptoms.

Finding a cause is not as simple as it may sound. As a matter of fact, doctors often go through the process of ruling out serious disorders, eventually reaching the point where they can tell you what you don't have but they can't exactly tell you what you do have. This usually means that it probably is nothing serious and you can live with it for a while and it will probably go away. They don't have to do anything about it because if there is a change in your symptoms you'll come back.

Because medicine is not an exact science, the doctor cannot diagnose and then treat a disorder simply by running a few tests and pushing a few buttons. Resolving complicated or mysterious disorders can be frustrating not only to your doctor but also to you as a pilot. You are used to immediately correcting something that goes wrong. Your emergency checklist considers every conceivable cause of a problem and gives you an immediate solution. Not so in medicine. It can take days, weeks, or even months to thoroughly evaluate and treat your disorder. This may be very difficult for you to accept, and you are tempted by your equally anxious colleagues to take inappropriate courses of action to hurry up the process. This understandable situation can only lead to a more difficult conclusion that eventually will have to be explained to the FAA.

A doctor often practices defensive medicine, doing more tests than necessary and treating aggressively to avoid overlooking a disease, making a misdiagnosis, or being accused of malpractice. You may even expect, and often demand, that additional testing be done to get back your medical certification. Nevertheless, the doctor works toward a goal of diagnosis and therapy by first ruling out serious conditions, often coming up with the diagnosis, and then getting on with taking care of the symptoms (which you saw the doctor for in the first place). In any case, the nonpilot patient can go back to work during this evaluation and treatment period.

If there is a change or if you don't get any better, you return to the doctor. This is an ongoing process of evaluation, ruling out causes, and treatment until the symptoms go away or a more definitive diagnosis is made along with a specific, curative treatment. The difference between private and FAA practice is that the private doctor is trying to find the causes of the symptoms of an unhealthy population and then treat the patients for long-term health and the FAA is trying to prove the absence of disease in a usually healthy population until the next required exam.

SATISFYING FAA REQUIREMENTS

This whole process is meant to keep you healthy, and if your own family doctor is comfortable with your health and medical care, why isn't the FAA? The biggest difference is that the FAA looks at your health as something that should not change in the near future, usually six to twelve months from the time you are examined. The FAA knows full well that you will not come running to your AME if there is a change in your medical status. Therefore, the AME must determine, at the time of your physical, if you have a medical problem or are likely to develop one and what its impact is on safe flight.

If you have symptoms that an AME finds potentially disqualifying, it must be determined that the data does not represent a problem for flying now or in the immediate future. This determination requires a more extensive evaluation—probably more of an evaluation than your own doctor would find necessary. You are reluctant to divulge too much information for fear that something will turn up, and a doctor will be the first one to admit that, if enough tests are done, a problem will be found.

So what happens with these results? With the nonflying patient, the doctor will probably treat the problem or just observe for weeks and months. The

FAA, however, knows that it can't monitor you on a daily or weekly basis, so it requires more data to confirm that your present good health will continue. The evaluation necessary to provide these data may not be medically justified to most nonaviation doctors. Therefore, you are caught between two types of medical evaluation standards: a set of results that could ground you and standards that would be medically acceptable to your family doctor. There is also a third standard—you may not feel that the problem is disqualifying.

In the new FAA medical regulations of September 1996, there is no blood pressure standard; that is, there are no longer regulation "numbers" with which to gauge your level of hypertension or high blood pressure. Recognizing that blood pressure is very dynamic and merely having your blood pressure taken in your AME's office is enough to make it go up, the FAA has chosen to leave the diagnosis of hypertension (persistent elevated blood pressure) up to the examining physician or AME. That diagnosis will be judged very differently by different doctors, so it is imperative that you are familiar with what we are discussing here.

A commonly held view is that the tests doctors use and how they treat patients is their responsibility and that they will take appropriate measures to keep patients healthy. They are working without having to answer to a government bureaucracy. Even if the process takes several weeks or months, the typical patient can still work.

This may not be true for you as a pilot, however, since the FAA must ensure that your disorder, the test results, and your therapy will not interfere with your flying responsibilities now and in the future, something your private doctor doesn't usually need to consider. Consequently, the FAA may require you to have more data to establish your present and potential health, data your family doctor (and insurance company) may not feel are required. Therefore, coupled with data gathered by your doctor, all of this information may be more than is realistically necessary to prove your health. Usually, the data would not have been needed at all if you had known what to do to keep healthy.

REASONABLE AND ACCEPTABLE STANDARDS

You can now understand the dilemma. What your own doctor would do in your own best medical interests may not coincide with what the FAA needs, and you certainly don't want to be grounded. Your doctor may feel that your disorder is perfectly safe to fly with, yet if your doctor knew about the physiology of flying, he or she would know the disorder could be risky.

By the same token, the FAA may accept a medical condition without a lot of extensive evaluation and treatment as long as it does not create a problem in the months to come. Also, the FAA may accept a disorder that your own doctor wouldn't, especially if your doctor is somewhat afraid of flying. For example, the FAA will accept a blood pressure level that your own doctor would

consider too high. In contrast, as I stated earlier, the FAA may want more information about a problem than your own doctor feels is necessary.

Remember, two of the tools that your family doctor can use are "tincture
of time" and observation, but the FAA must have immediate and current objective data with which to judge your flying status now and until the next exam.
Your own doctor may feel that there is no reason why you can't fly, but your
doctor probably doesn't know that your problem could be unsafe. I have seen
many reports from well-meaning physicians stating that in their judgment you,
the patient, can fly when in fact the problem is a potential threat to safe flying.
This conclusion is confusing to the unknowing pilot.

Thus, the triple standard: yours, your doctor's, and the FAA's (and you
could even add the additional standards of your colleagues, company, and family).

THE REALITY OF A PILOT'S HEALTH

As discussed in Chapter 4, cardiovascular disease—high blood pressure and
coronary artery disease—is one of the most common causes of medical ground-
ings, although often this denial is ultimately overcome. In the case of increased
blood pressure, medication is often the treatment of choice, but this treatment
is also a direct threat to a pilot's career and medical certification.

Coronary artery disease is often viewed by a doctor as treatable simply
by a change in lifestyle (e.g., developing an exercise program or losing weight)
and the use of medication to control the disease and any complications. To a
pilot, merely having a history of significant coronary artery disease is a mandatory disqualification. If you have acquired this disorder, you are grounded as
soon as the diagnosis is made.

So what's my point? If you are ill or notice symptoms that you haven't
had before (assuming you are in excellent health to begin with), you must work
with your family doctor so that, in addition to caring for your health, he or she
understands your minimum flying requirements. Be sure that your doctor does
not become overly aggressive in evaluation or therapy but does enough to obtain adequate information if the FAA requires it.

Remember that your doctor probably knows little about the FAA and its
procedures and probably even less about how your medical condition and the
effects of therapy will impact your ability to fly safely. He or she could be a
"white knuckler" and overly protective about your flying health or may "allow"
you to continue flying when, in the judgment of the FAA and a qualified
aeromedical physician, your condition would not be compatible with safe flying. Keep in mind that your personal doctor is *not* the one to determine if you
are certifiable.

An interesting question is whether or not doctors could tell pilots too much. An analogy would be whether or not a pilot should tell passengers that an engine has been lost, even though they are in no danger and they will not have to turn back. The passengers may expect to be informed, but is this information in the best interests of the passengers, especially if they don't understand the ramifications? Many will say that it's best to inform the passengers, but that requires a great deal of tact.

Therefore, be sure your doctor doesn't tag you in the medical record with too many possible diagnoses. The record may come back to haunt you if it is not discretely defined at the time of the diagnosis. I am not advocating ignoring a medical problem or stating that it should not be corrected. But knowing that there is this dilemma, it is quite frustrating to me to realize that the majority of the medical disorders that ground a pilot could not only be corrected and controlled but actually prevented if the pilot would follow commonsense health maintenance, understand the certification process, and trust professional people. I realize that most pilots will not be concerned about their health until something goes wrong, but crisis management doesn't protect pilots' health or medical certification.

PERCEPTIONS OF FAA AND COMPANY DOCTORS

I would like to make a comment here regarding a relatively common feeling among some pilots in commercial aviation. There is a notion, especially among some of the "leaders" of the pilot community and some publications, that not only is the FAA out to get pilots but so is the company employing them. This attitude is fortunately the exception, not the rule. Still, this rumor discredits the works of some company aviation doctors and dedicated private practice aviation doctors who truly are on the pilot's side.

Doctors must play by the rules of scientific, factual medicine. Their critics, however, don't need to follow these rules because they are not responsible for your health and safety. A doctor can't necessarily resolve a problem in a matter of hours. This is not the result of inefficiency. Whether you like the doctor's findings or not, he or she is still the only one who knows about your true health. Would you accept the comments of a friend over those of a professional mechanic when dealing with the performance of your aircraft?

Everybody loses if you don't fly, including the airline, your company, and your family. To put the "doctors are out to get you" philosophy in a pilot's mind is unfair because the pilot may want a doctor's assistance in the future. Unfounded comments are an injustice to the pilot with a career at stake. At least check out the other side of the stories you hear.

Usually if a pilot is medically grounded by the company doctor, aviation doctor, or FAA, it is for a valid reason, a reason not often shared with the rest of the world. The outsiders pass judgment based upon what they hear: "Joe couldn't possibly be sick enough to ground—the doc must be incompetent." Or worse: "Jolene is a great pilot, and there are pilots out there who are in worse shape. There's no reason why she shouldn't be flying." This, in my estimation, does a gross disservice to the pilot community and to the doctors trying to keep flight crews flying.

Remember, the doctor is only the messenger of bad news. You are the one who has the abnormal condition, not the doctor. The doctor can't simply ignore it. Furthermore, extensive evaluation for medical certification isn't necessary unless there is a reason to do more tests. The FAA, not the doctor, developed the guidelines that determined that Jolene's medical problem made her a flight risk.

There is a way to control your health and medical certification. Find out about your health and keep healthy. Know how the FAA certifies pilots. Find an aeromedical physician who is knowledgeable—one that you can trust—then stick with him or her. You don't have to rely on rumors to guide you if you know what to expect. Keep ahead of your health and certification. That way you can avoid a premature and incomplete report to the FAA.

Your challenge for protecting that medical certificate should now be clear—keep healthy and hang onto your medical certificate without making waves with the FAA. Meeting this challenge is not that difficult because you do have control over your flying career.

Therefore, check up on your family doctor and AME. Do they really understand your requirements? Is the AME a pilot? What does the AME do with the medical reports—does he or she send them immediately to the FAA? How active is the AME in the professional organizations that promote knowledge in general medicine and aerospace medicine?

I encourage you to become more familiar with the FAA's standards, expectations, and procedures. Don't expect your family doctor to understand that without a medical certificate you are permanently "disabled" or grounded. Communicate this to your family doctor or trusted AME and actually work with the FAA to protect your certificate.

If there still is doubt in your mind whether your doctor is adequately evaluating or overevaluating, whether he or she is overtreating or undertreating, or if your health could affect your career, you might consider calling Oklahoma City or your Regional Flight Surgeon and, without using your name, ask for advice. If you know of a knowledgeable AME or have an aeromedical consultant, call this person. If you don't know an aeromedical doctor, then find one who is known and respected by the FAA. The FAA considers recommendations from these doctors as very important. In addition, I am sure that your own doctor would be glad to know what to do or not to do since he or she is looking out for your future as well as for your health.

Also remember to tell your personal doctor that he or she is not responsible for making the determination that you are legal and fit to fly. That's the job of the FAA. Your doctor's role is just to provide information to another doctor in the FAA.

If there is no reason to distrust your company aviation doctor or AME, keep him or her informed. This person could be your strongest ally in protecting your medical certificate. An AME can't help you if you don't share how you are feeling and what is going on with your own family doctor. Of all the pilots who have followed this philosophy, perhaps 1 percent have not benefitted, but you won't hear about the 99 percent who were helped. You must put your trust in somebody. With so much at stake—not only your health but also your career and medical certificate—assume, unless you know or are sure otherwise, that the company doctor or aviation doctor is truly on your side and is anxious to help you. The "pink and breathing" exam of some AMEs may be the least threatening, but it also will give you a false sense of security.

If you still wish to see your private doctor for maintaining your health and then your AME for certification, that's fine. Just be sure that your private doctor knows that you are a pilot and that your AME will cooperate if anything abnormal is found. What you learn in this book will be an adequate guide to help both doctors. As mentioned before, if there is any doubt about the status of your health, ground yourself but seek help from a competent AME or from the FAA anonymously. Don't depend upon aeromedically uninformed doctors who can create more problems. Check with those who truly know.

Better still, know the status of your health and practice a good health maintenance program so you don't get caught behind the power curve.

IN REVIEW

1. Know and understand the process of certification and how medical disorders affect your flying and consequently your certificate.

2. Find that AME or private doctor who has good credentials, is active in aviation and aviation medicine, and is willing to take the time and effort to work with you. Do it now, not when you're grounded.

3. Make informed judgments about this AME or private doctor; don't make judgments based on hearsay or rumors from disgruntled pilots. Ask pilots if they can recommend AMEs. Judge the AME or private doctor based on the issues discussed in this chapter. Does the doctor know what to do? Has the doctor evaluated a pilot before, and what will he or she do if you have a medical problem? Does the doctor know what additional information the FAA will need if a disorder is found?

4. If there is any doubt about your disorder being prematurely reported to the FAA, tell your doctor or AME that you will not fly. That is, you will ground yourself until the problem is resolved and a report to the FAA can be deferred. A report to the FAA can then be made when you are ready.

5. Before your doctor puts you on medicine that you could be taking for

an extended period, be sure that there are no other ways to control your problem, such as diet, exercise, or stress management.

6. Show your doctor what your medical certification requirements are, and if you don't think your doctor understands, ask him or her to call the FAA or a professional aeromedical physician.

7. Take it upon yourself to practice good health maintenance so you don't get caught in the middle.

8. If you know of a problem that may be initially disqualifying, refer back to Chapter 3 for the specifics on preserving your medical certificate. Also check Appendix II.

Remember, the issue is whether or not you are medically safe to fly. Do you have a condition that could unpredictably impair you tomorrow? Your proficiency and experience flying, unfortunately, have no bearing on your fitness to fly. You must accept that ultimate responsibility, and you may have to educate your doctor and your AME so they can be more supportive.

6

A Pilot's Own Health Maintenance Program

A forty-six-year-old corporate pilot was overweight, out of shape, and cared little about her self-image. Her husband was not in ideal health either. Fortunately (or unfortunately), she passed her FAA exam without problems and had little incentive to change her lifestyle. However, a grounded pilot did get her attention by explaining that she also did not take her health seriously and was suddenly grounded because of increased blood pressure. The pilot and her husband reevaluated their priorities. They both got back into shape and now actually enjoy being active in their free time.

Look back to your introduction to IFR flying and how you watched, with awe, the "real" pilot break out of the clouds and land right down the middle of the runway approach lights. And then you attempted to do it. You quickly found that flying an aircraft was one thing, but flying the gauges, communicating with ATC, and reading approach plates added a seemingly overwhelming burden to even the most professional pilot. But you finally got it together, and you realized that most of what you now were doing—flying IFR—was by habit. You didn't have to think out everything that you had to do. How did this learning happen?

If you recall, you first read books. Then you had someone show you how IFR works, and then you practiced what you read and what you were shown. And you continue to do this to this day. The proof of your success is passing the periodic check ride. Learning is one thing, reinforcement of key topics is another and no less important.

Developing your own health maintenance program is similar. You can't expect to do this without preparation any more than you can learn to fly the ILS back course only by watching your instructor. Your doctor can't make you follow a program—he or she has no magic pills. Your doctor can't get you out of the trouble that you brought upon yourself with abuses to your health.

So the first thing you must do is to learn about the regulations that concern your health. You can't assume that the doctor knows these regulations any more or less than you. This is particularly true for the September 1996 revisions to the FAA medical standards because they represent a change in how the FAA looks at your medical certification. New technology and new evaluations of the risk of specific medical disorders give you more latitude to maintain your certificate. In addition, you must recognize the expectations of the FAA and your company regarding your fitness to fly and medical certification.

Then you must learn your true health status by having a good medical evaluation from a doctor who also knows the rules. Some will say that a regular physical is unnecessary, and for some people, it might be. But professional pilots must not only be healthy when they're at the controls, they must protect their careers and medical certificates by staying healthy. They must maintain a lifestyle that is consistent throughout the years. They must take physicals to keep ahead. Ideally, they should have a medical preflight exam every time they fly, but that's totally unrealistic and wouldn't be in the best interest of pilots (even though there are countries that do a mini-exam prior to every major trip). Health care should be like the preventive maintenance of aircraft. Like the evaluation of your flying in dual training, an evaluation of your health must be done by someone you can trust and respect. This must be someone who does not feel the FAA must be immediately notified if you are less than in perfect health.

THE COMPLETE MEDICAL EVALUATION AND RISK FACTORS

The health maintenance evaluation should include a thorough physical exam, a chest X ray (if there is a clinical need such as a history of smoking), a resting ECG, blood and urine tests, breathing tests, a test for blood in your bowel movements, and the usual vision and hearing tests. The most important part of any medical evaluation is a comprehensive, confidential medical history. Patients rarely share a candid history, especially if the doctor is an AME. Still, this history is vitally important to the doctor's evaluation.

From this exam, you determine your risk factors, factors that could statistically increase your risk of developing medical problems and decrease your chances of keeping your medical certificate. You can't correct faults that lead to increased risk until you identify them. What is your cholesterol level? Has your ECG changed? Are you overweight and out of shape?

If your doctor identifies risk factors, you can practice correcting them until you are sure that you can pass your next physical without fear because you have developed good health habits.

By identifying your risk factors and trying to correct them, you begin to determine what factors keep you from achieving your goal—your perfect medical check ride. Is it habit and lack of self-control or is it too much temptation that keeps those risk factors ever present? So how do you improve that over-correcting tendency on the glide slope? By the same technique for learning good health habits—practice and patience. There is no shortcut to health maintenance or to maintaining flying proficiency.

Maybe you have identified your risk factors, but you have been unable to correct them although you've tried many times. Why? You certainly are motivated. You know what has to be done, but you don't progress the way the books say you should. You continue to gain weight, and you still smoke and drink too much. You haven't gotten around to committing to an exercise program, and you rationalize that "as long as I feel good—not to worry." But you do worry when you take your FAA exam.

CONTROLLING RISK FACTORS

The solution should be apparent. But you can't do it alone, and you can't do it without changing old habits first. That means working with your doctor and his or her assistants, giving them time to explain what needs to be done, and then practicing and returning, practicing and returning, practicing and returning. You may have to tell the doctor what your special aeromedical needs are, but your doctor knows the medical part.

Find out what the ideal health of a pilot should be. Talk to others who have licked the same problem you need to. Don't depend upon techniques that are not generally accepted. Get the facts. Rarely has any part of health maintenance really changed much over the years. Stick to your plan but remember that few people have been able to do it alone. A pilot's pride is no less than a doctor's, and I know it is hard for doctors to let go of old ideas. Doctors' egos sometimes get in the way of logical health maintenance. Remember, though, I can go back to work with an illness.

When considering claims for a "new and revolutionary" diet or health maintenance program, which may not be generally accepted or proven useful by the medical profession, remember that a promoter of this program is not obligated to discuss the pros and cons. Doctors, on the other hand, must advise you of their recommendations. After all, they are ultimately responsible for your health; others don't have that accountability. Doctors can do this only after considering all sides of the issue, both pro and con, and their advice must be tailored to your individual requirements. In other words, if John Doe advertises a new program for better health, he will use only those studies and testimonials that will further his cause. He will not use any reports that could dispute his claim. Beware of claims that use the words "astonishing results," "newly discovered," and "remarkable program."

Now, if Doctor Jane Doe is asked what she thinks of a particular program, she is obligated, in your best interest, to share all sides of the claimed benefits.

She may appear negative, which adds to the frustration of the pilot looking for a good program, especially one that is reported to be a quick fix. What to do? Consider the source, the program's reputation, and whether you know the cons as well as the pros. No program is free of cons. Look to your own doctor for advice; don't play doctor. Your family and friends are poor medical consultants.

We all are inherently impatient and want to see results in a matter of days or weeks. When we don't see a change right away, we become discouraged and slip back into our old, comfortable, unchallenging habits. We don't modify our health by simply studying our problems and not taking action—or, worse, bouncing back and forth between programs.

CHANGING HABITS

You now know what is expected of you by the FAA. You also are—or should be—working with a doctor who knows your health status and recognizes the limitations put on you by the FAA and your flying responsibilities. As a result, you have identified your risk factors and have made an attempt to identify the elements controlling them. For example, you are overweight and your cholesterol and triglycerides are up and your HDL is down. You have recorded your intake in a diary so you know where the extra calories and fatty foods are coming from. You talk with your spouse and discuss your need to modify the meals you eat together. But what about when you are on a trip? Those flight lunches leave a lot to be desired. What do you order when you go out to eat? Go back to the basics described in Chapter 7. Who says you can't brown bag your meals? Who says you have to clean your plate?

But the motivation will get weaker unless you really have changed that old lifestyle. This gets us into the hardest part of doing that: how to maintain the drive that keeps everything under control.

Try different tricks. Tack a copy of your medical certificate and a chart of goals on the refrigerator door or on the mirror in the bathroom to remind you to eat right and to exercise. Find a buddy with the same problem and support each other. Return to your doctor's office for monitoring. Sure it is expensive and a nuisance, but it beats sitting at home grounded.

THE PILOT'S RESPONSIBILITY IN HEALTH MAINTENANCE

Earlier in the book, I expressed my feelings about the pass the buck philosophy of some AMEs. This may be your philosophy, too, because many pilots who fail at health maintenance want to blame someone else. A favorite "cover your rear end" statement by people promoting a new diet or health aid that may not work is "ask your doctor." Well, your doctor can't help you either if you don't practice discipline. If you approach a health maintenance program as you would cramming for an exam and then discontinue good health maintenance practices after the FAA exam, you are jeopardizing your career, even though you passed the test. Anyone can pass an exam by cramming. I frequently see pilots who schedule their flight physicals during times of the year when they know they have better control of their weight or exercise program.

Many professional pilots have much of their flying career spelled out for them by FARs and company policies, and some have a lot of the mundane parts of flying done for them, such as filing flight plans and obtaining weather reports. This allows the pilots to concentrate on flying, but it also gives them a false sense of "who is responsible" for other matters dealing with their careers, especially their medical certificates. They become complacent because they expect others to do work for them. I hope that by now you realize no one but you is responsible for your health. The FAA and your company screen out unhealthy flight crew members who could be responsible for an accident, but you are responsible for not being one of those who allowed their poor health to interfere with their careers.

Unlike most other aspects of professional flying, your medical status and how you maintain your health are purely up to you. You picked a career that requires your good health be proven to a government agency. By staying healthy and understanding the certification process, there is very little chance of your being unnecessarily grounded. I have stated it many times, and I will state it once more: don't let the FAA be the one to tell you to do the things you should be doing anyway to remain a healthy and safe pilot. Many times I have encouraged pilots to no avail to improve their health. They do finally lose their medical certificates, and to be recertified, it takes months of getting back into shape and considerable anguish and frustration. Looking back, pilots will usually admit that the FAA forced them into changing their habits. Prior planning could have prevented that disruption in their careers.

IN REVIEW

The keys to the success of your health maintenance program are knowing what has to be done and why as well as working with someone who can be very objective about your program. Let's review the steps:

1. Know your obligations and restrictions by being familiar with FAR Part 67, "Medical Standards and Certification," with special emphasis on the 1996 revisions.

2. Fully understand and be comfortable with the meaning of FAR 61.53, especially the strategy of grounding yourself so that you do not have to immediately report a problem to the FAA.

3. Know your true health and identify risk factors by having a periodic, thorough medical evaluation by a doctor who knows your requirements and restrictions.

4. Under the supervision of your doctor, change your old habits and learn healthier ones.

5. Tell your doctor about your obligations to the FAA. Be sure your doctor or his or her assistants are willing and able to help you in your ongoing health maintenance program.

6. Finally, keep on top of your health status, just as you do your flying status. Keep working toward your goals. If one way doesn't work, try another but only after you gave the former a good try. There are no quick fixes. Do whatever it takes to get the job done. Monitor yourself continuously and have someone keep score for you.

This monitoring need not require fancy tests or frequent returns to your doctor or therapist. Measurements you can take and record will be an excellent guide to how you are progressing. These include how your clothes fit, your pulse rate at rest and with exercise, your weight, the measurement of your waist and biceps, how you are sleeping (are you rested in the morning?), and what belt holes you are using (hang your belt up every night so you can see it). You might even consider taking a picture of yourself once a month so that you can compare the photographs. And look to your spouse (and children) for candid but caring monitoring.

7

Airworthy Anatomy *by Sharon M. Hanks*

A forty-three-year old airline pilot had a problem with weight. She just couldn't lose more than a few pounds without gaining them back. Over the years, her blood pressure rose. She became a ping-pong dieter, going on crash diets prior to her FAA exam and then allowing the fat to return. Eventually, her blood pressure reached a consistently elevated state regardless of her weight. She's flying, but she's under constant monitoring by the FAA even though she finally has her weight under control.

Even under a deluge of duties, demands, decisions, and dangers, pilots are expected to function with optimum efficiency at all times. The level of responsibility involved in expertly maneuvering airplanes and safely transporting thousands of lives is very high—it requires pilots to function without error. They must exhibit the utmost mental capability, extreme emotional stability, and excellent physical condition to meet the superhuman expectations of those around them—the passengers and public as well as the FAA and their company.

Certainly, you would expect that pilots would do absolutely everything in their power to safeguard the workings of their intricate human machines, for their careers depend upon the premise of good health. But it seems as though pilots often give more attention to the health of their aircraft than to the health of their bodies. Pilots would never consider going on a trip without having enough fuel aboard their airplanes, but ironically, they are willing to begin the day's journey without enough fuel in their bodies—without having eaten an adequate meal. Pilots know that it would be foolish to expect a 747 to execute a successful takeoff burning gasohol, and yet at times they try to squeeze their essential minimum daily requirements out of a dozen cups of coffee and a sweet roll. They also seek to prevent any possible mechanical failure by conducting thorough preflight exams while, in contrast, their own bodily gauges and indicators of impending physical failure go unnoticed or disregarded. In reality, however, even pilots are not immune to the human shortcomings of im-

---

Sharon M. Hanks was Dr. Richard Reinhart's medical assistant and educational director. She has a B.S. degree in health care science.

proper eating and activities that can have devastating effects on maintaining their airworthy anatomies and careers.

Eating sensibly is vital to maintaining excellent health and physical fitness. This applies to everyone: young and old, male, and female, rich and poor. You probably have heard the phrase, "you are what you eat." Obviously, what you are is not limited only to what you eat. What you are as a person is also influenced by what you see, hear, read, know, and experience. And, of course, it depends on your genes. But speaking in terms of the physical body, what you are is, most commonly, what goes into the stomach. That rich, red blood that flows to the far reaches of the body, hastening the emergency oxygen rations to deficient, suffocating cells when you soar at high altitudes, those sturdy bones comprising your frame that support your movements and allow you to board and operate the aircraft, those delicate brain cells that miraculously spark every instantaneous thought, every crucial cockpit calculation—all of these, and virtually every single cell of your body, are formed and maintained by using the vital substances gleaned from the foods (or unfoods) that you eat. The importance of the quality of your food should be quite obvious. But, in spite of the apparent significance, getting all of the proper kinds of food fuel for the body, in the correct amounts, is all too often overlooked.

The problems associated with food and nutrition are very different today than they were centuries ago. The problem for people in the past was to provide enough food for themselves and their family for subsistence. People had to battle nature to grow their own crops and raise their own livestock. They suffered from all kinds of dietary deficiencies and natural diseases. In contrast, food and nutrition problems in the United States today are just the opposite. Food is overly abundant, available, and appealing. Our problem is eating too much and yet too poorly for a well-balanced diet. No longer do we "eat to live"; the emphasis is now becoming "live to eat." No longer do we struggle to satisfy hunger; instead we indulge the appetite. (Furthermore, unique to flying, hunger does frequently become the sole sense we need to satisfy through any means available.) It is estimated that 30–50 percent of the population of the United States is obese.

By the way, the term *obese* includes such states as being *pleasingly plump, roly-poly,* and *slightly overweight,* terms that are used to make light of a seriously heavy situation. We continue to eat ourselves to death, literally. It has become a way of life.

Ironically, at the same time that Americans boast of technological accomplishments, advancements in medical science, great strides in food production, and an ever-increasing knowledge of nutrition, this country is faced with epidemic proportions of nutritionally related degenerative problems like heart disease, atherosclerosis, hypertension, stroke, diabetes, obesity, and anemias. We are proud because we are so rich and food is so abundant, but heart disease continues to be our number one killer. We consume a disproportionate percentage of the world's available foodstuffs while trying—unsuccessfully—to ignore the consequences of being overweight. We hardly know the meaning of scarcity, starvation, or famine. Some countries don't know the meaning of heart disease, atherosclerosis, and obesity!

The abuse of food accompanied by the neglect of physical activity has placed us in the midst of a coronary epidemic, where we are forced to deal with diseases that we can't blame on the invasion of microorganisms. We can't pass the buck to infection by innocent bacteria or viruses. Instead, we have brought a plague upon ourselves by our own mistakes, apathy, affluence, and unwillingness to listen to the advice of those who are trying desperately to help. People are always willing to listen and change their ways after having had a heart attack—provided they survive it. It is unfortunate that it takes such a drastic and painful measure to arouse their interest. It is especially disastrous for pilots, who not only jeopardize their health but also potentially lose their careers in the process.

The American lifestyle verges on gluttony. We eat very rich foods with empty calories in infinite quantities while our activity level is dangerously low. Consumption of fat-laden meats and dairy products has been on the rise while purchase of valuable, vitamin-rich fruits, vegetables, and grains has diminished. Our frenzied pace has encouraged more frequent use of restaurants, especially the fast-food type. We also are relying more on heavily processed junk foods. Hard physical labor has given way to sedentary desk work. Driving has replaced that valuable means of transportation, walking. The use of leisure time in recreation and sports has been undermined by the art of gawking at the tube for hours on end, with all too frequent trips to the refrigerator.

The eventual consequences of all of this physical idleness and overeating to our heart's content—or, more accurately, at our heart's expense—are unavoidable but controllable. If not brought under control, these bad habits soon can force you to become a mere statistic in the national mortality tables. Fortunately, you can employ a better lifestyle, one of prudent eating and exercise, and work toward the prevention of heart disease and diabetes. You can reduce your risk of heart disease and its associated diseases and possibly even reverse the degenerative process to some extent. So don't just sit back like a time bomb ready to explode and wait for some warning. By the time symptoms of heart disease or diabetes appear, the insidious illness has already progressed far. Sometimes the near-fatal heart attack is the first and ultimate warning! And then no physician's good intentions, no miracle drug, no magic wand, no sum of money, and no amount of fame can mend that neglected heart. The time to act is now, just when you think you don't need to act.

Every human being has the instinct to survive. We all desire a long, healthy, and happy life. Our bodies are supposed to last—they were made that way—to be strong and not break down during prime years. High blood pressure, diabetes, a stroke, and heart problems should not prematurely halt your most productive years. Pilots are supposed to reach sixty and well beyond. Unlike some other machines, the human machine improves with use. Inactivity only causes degradation. Sensible eating, accompanied by vigorous physical activity, is essential to optimal health and longevity. This is no big surprise. So why do so many people still face serious health problems?

In recent years nutritional controversies have saturated the media, causing much confusion. You undoubtedly have been bombarded with articles about nutritional cults, food faddists, miracle diets, the harmful effects of table sugar, cholesterol and heart disease, additives and preservatives, yogurt as a cure-all, health food stores, megavitamins, and many, many more health-related topics. Further complicating the matter is the power of Madison Avenue ads capable of selling any product, good or bad. The health food/weight loss business is a mutimillion-dollar industry preying on you and me, making it very difficult to know the truth about sensible eating. It is my intention to weed through the cluttered media mess for you in order to salvage some facts.

Actually, some of the very basic rules of a sound diet have not changed much over the years. Their age does not make them invalid, just as popularity does not guarantee credibility. Therefore, don't be too quick to discard rules that you learned years ago and to latch onto new ones. Instead, be informed so that you can distinguish the beneficial suggestions from the useless or harmful. Incorporate new findings gradually and intelligently so that the important ideas become a permanent part of your life and not merely a brief fling.

THE FUEL

When it comes to eating, why do you choose that substance commonly known as food? Why not have a bowl of gravel with a side order of wood shavings to get your minerals and fiber?

The main reason for eating a meal in the first place is to consume the foods that contain all of the necessary ingredients to provide the cells of the body with the supplies for energy, building, and repair. This is your main thought while perusing a menu of delectables in your favorite French restaurant, right? Ridiculous! The act of eating has become more complex. If procuring nutrients were the only consideration, our dining habits would be quite primitive.

Fortunately, but unfortunately for some abusers, eating has become a much more complex, social activity. Eating is a pleasurable, satisfying experience. Food entices the senses with visual appeal, savory aromas, assorted textures, and a spectrum of flavors. Mealtime is an important part of home life and family togetherness. Eating is a pleasant part of daily living around which many social and business gatherings are planned. Eating habits have cultural qualities and great national diversity. Some foods have deep religious symbolism. All of our cherished holidays and traditions are centered around foods of particular significance. Even the changing seasons influence our eating; we anticipate the foods that make their limited annual appearance. Consider also the phenomenon of munching, a casual perversion of conscious, intelligent ingestion that goes hand-in-hand (or hand-to-mouth) with spectator sports and movies.

Obviously, our selection of foods should be based largely on the actual content of products and how they benefit our bodies. But many subconscious factors negatively influence our decisions and may jeopardize our health. It is important to be knowledgeable about food facts while being aware of subconscious forces, both good and bad, in order to remain in control of your intake.

So what is food, anyway? Take a moment to scrutinize it. See that buffet table heaped with beautifully prepared gourmet delights, colorful arrangements of luscious chef's masterpieces, and exquisite, rare delicacies? A gorgeous sight—better than crew meals! Try to think about needs for a moment instead of wants, as impossible as that seems in this situation. Remember that there is more to food than tastes, smells, and a distended abdomen. Nutrition is the process by which the substances that you eat become you. What you eat today flies the plane tomorrow! The nutrient part of that food is really what your body is seeking. And you can find it even at the smorgasbord if you look past the frills and embellishments, around the garnishes and decorations, and through the marinades and sauces. Food is dressed up and camouflaged with infinite variety, but if you zoom in for a microscopic view, you find that each dish consists of the same minute building blocks, or nutrients. Everything from the chateaubriand to the chocolate mousse can be broken down into six essential kinds of nutrients—proteins, carbohydrates, fats, vitamins, minerals, and water. Stack the building blocks one way and you have a pork chop. Stack them another way, and you've got a string bean.

Nutrients are actually chemical substances, arrangements of atoms into complex molecules, naturally occurring in foods, that work together and interact with body chemicals. They are essential for building, operation, and repair of body tissue, for efficient functioning, and for furnishing fuel. Each nutrient has a specific use in the body. No one natural food, by itself, contains all the required nutrients. Many kinds and combinations of foods together can lead to a well-balanced diet. Therefore, you need a variety of foods each day to ensure that you are getting all the different, necessary nutrients. Everyone needs the same nutrients throughout life but in different amounts depending on factors such as age, sex, activity level, occupation, environmental stress, size, state of health, and pregnancy.

Every single bite that you take at each meal and in between has to be processed by your body and affects your body immediately and cumulatively. Your body has to deal with every particle of that delicious T-bone that you had last night while on layover as well as every additive in that hotdog that you just inhaled during the last brief stop. Don't think that you can eat something just for the fun of it and that it then will simply pass right through you and out. Having a piece of pie à la mode after a huge banquet doesn't mean that the pie won't have any effect on your system. Something has to be done with it, even though you didn't need it. Your body either will use it or store it (and you know where) along with the extras from yesterday and the day before and the day before that. Get the picture?

Long after you chow down, your digestive system is hard at work processing the food and breaking it down into nutrients or nutrient combinations and waste products. Your blood, which continually circulates, absorbs nutrients from the digestive tract and oxygen from the lungs and carries them to each cell in the body. Some of the essential nutrients need to be replenished every day. Others can be stored for future use, but an excess of one can never compensate for a shortage of another. Sometimes certain nutrients are only effective when working together as teams. For example, in building bones, the nutrients vitamin D, calcium, and phosphorus must interact. One member of the team cannot perform its job unless all the others are present in the right proportions. Thus, variety of foods and moderation in amount are two key concepts in a wise eating pattern.

PROTEIN

Protein is required by all living things. It is the basic substance making up every cell of the body and is needed by everyone throughout life for many important functions:

- Building and maintaining body tissues
- Rapid tissue growth in the womb and during childhood
- Recovering after excess destruction or loss, such as burns, surgery, hemorrhage, and infection
- Making hemoglobin, which carries oxygen to the cells and carbon dioxide away
- Making up the part of the DNA molecule that carries the genetic code
- Producing thousands of enzymes, which control the chemical reactions of the body
- Producing hormones, which regulate body processes
- Supplying energy in shortage situations
- Regulating water balance and the acid-base balance

Protein is made up of smaller chemical units called "amino acids." During digestion the proteins from foods are broken down into amino acids, which are then rearranged into different proteins for special functions in the human body. There are twenty or more different amino acids, which serve as building blocks of proteins. The protein molecules resemble long chains where each link is an amino acid chemically joined by peptide bonds. Each protein molecule has hundreds of amino acids linked into long chains in an endless number of combinations and sequences, making possible an almost infinite variety of proteins.

The body can synthesize most of the amino acids from foods, but some must be provided ready-made in the diet. They are known as "essential" amino acids. There are eight: lysine, tryptophan, methionine, phenylalanine, threonine, valine, leucine, and isoleucine. Food proteins providing all of the essential amino acids in the amounts and proportions needed by the body are known as "complete" proteins and rate highest in quality. A low-value protein lacks one or more of the indispensable amino acids and cannot support life by itself. However, two different proteins with limiting amino acids may complement each other and together provide a higher value.

Animal products—meat, fish, poultry, milk, cheese, and eggs—are high-quality proteins and are sources of readily available essential amino acids. Animal body composition is similar to that of humans, and thus animal proteins supply more of the essential amino acids than plant foods. Fruits, vegetables, legumes, and grains are lower in quality because some amino acids are missing. Higher-quality protein foods can be teamed with lower-quality to provide good total protein nutrition when eaten together. The missing amino acids can be "filled in" to improve the overall balance. Some examples of teams are breakfast cereal with milk, rice with fish, macaroni with cheese, and spaghetti with meat sauce.

Some nutrients can be stored in the body for later use, but protein cannot. It must be supplied in the diet every day. It is best used when consumed in small amounts every few hours. Protein deficiency is not a major problem today in the United States. In fact, most of us eat much more protein than we need. This is biologically and economically wasteful. But we like lots of meat, and since we can afford to, we continue to consume large quantities of it, especially beef and pork. Years ago we used to rely heavily on the vegetable and grain sources of protein, but today the majority of our protein is taken from the more expensive animal sources. We have decreased the consumption of vegetables and grains at the expense of losing some valuable substances, while our increased use of animal products, which are heavy with fats, has contributed to new health problems.

Some people still believe that they gain weight from eating too many carbohydrates or too many food fats. But too many proteins can do the same thing. When burned, the carbohydrates and fats supply most of the body's energy. When not enough calories are available from the carbohydrates and fats to meet the energy demand, then the body may use some of the extra free proteins for energy calories. But usually, excess proteins are converted to body fat. So you can actually become fat from eating excess calories in the protein form just as you can from eating too many carbohydrate calories or too many food fat calories. It is the surplus of calories that adds pounds, regardless of where they came from. Overindulging in top quality steak can add inches to the waistline just as well as too many gooey sweet rolls.

Another misconception about proteins is that great quantities are needed to build muscle mass and to better your athletic performance. Since meat is muscle, many coaches and athletes have believed that eating meat, especially red meat, would increase muscle mass and overall strength. Thick steaks have been approved for many training meals. Actually, only a small amount of additional protein is needed during athletic conditioning for developing muscles, and as stated earlier, any excess protein is converted to body fat. Eating a sixteen-ounce piece of beef does not mean that you will add ounces to your biceps, any more than eating hair would diminish a bald spot or eating brain would increase your smarts.

If you are disappointed by your image in the mirror, and you long for a Superman or Superwoman physique, don't start investing in magical protein-supplement concoctions. The key to having strong, bulging muscles is not consuming a mountain of protein but doing a heap of exercise. If your goal is to be muscle-bound, a well-planned, supervised program of exercise, especially isometrics and isotonics, will bring the desired dimensions. Because of an increased energy expenditure while exercising, extra calories will be needed. They should come from a balanced diet emphasizing carbohydrates and fats, not extra protein. It is the exercise that induces muscle strength and hypertrophy, not more protein. We cannot make more muscle fibers in our bodies—the number stays the same—but we can force the ones that we have to get bigger.

Before you get too entangled in your vanity, keep in mind that exercise for the sole purpose of building the skeletal muscles is fine and harmless to a certain extent. But all too often the one most important and vital muscle in the whole body, the heart, is neglected. Pumping iron does build muscle mass, but it does nothing for your heart muscle. The only reason to be muscle-bound is for aesthetic reasons; it has no real lasting purpose unless the heart is equally conditioned. Certain types of exercise do focus on strengthening the heart and greatly benefit your life in terms of overall health, physical endurance, and longevity. They are aerobic exercises, such as running, bicycling, swimming, and walking (see Chapter 8). It is the cardiovascular system that needs the attention; we don't seem to be dying from weak arms but weak hearts. You'll often find that the skinny woman who rides her bicycle to work every day has more cardiovascular endurance than Mr. or Ms. Muscle.

CARBOHYDRATES

Carbohydrates are chemical combinations of carbon, hydrogen, and oxygen.

In order to survive, all animals must eat plants that supply carbohydrates. Only plants contain chlorophyll, which enables them to make carbohydrates from the carbon dioxide in the air and water in the soil while using the energy from the sun. Plant foods provide carbohydrates in three main forms: starches, sugars, and celluloses (fiber).

Like proteins, carbohydrate molecules also resemble chains in structure, where each link is a sugar molecule. This is not the white sugar that you find on the kitchen table. A larger carbohydrate molecule, like starch, is a chain of the smaller, simpler sugars, which function as building blocks. All carbohydrates must be broken down by digestion into simple sugars to be used as a source of energy by body tissues. Glucose, commonly known as "blood sugar," is the form mainly used by the body's cells. Some complex carbohydrates, such as cellulose, cannot be broken down by digestion in humans, and when eaten they simply supply the roughage that is needed for proper elimination of solid wastes.

The major function of carbohydrates in the body is to furnish the fuel for energy to do work, whether it be the silent, ongoing, internal body processes or all-out physical exertion. Glucose is one of the most important fuels. It is the main source of energy for red blood cells and the central nervous system—your brain. Carbohydrates spare proteins from being used up for energy by fulfilling the energy needs themselves and thus saving proteins for more important jobs such as tissue building and repair. Carbohydrates also help in the use of fats.

The body draws energy from carbohydrates mainly by converting the simple glucose molecule to carbon dioxide and water. This is one of the most vital chemical reactions in biology. It is the very essence of transforming the starch from a wonderfully nutritious baked potato into the actual energy needed to win a tennis match, fly an airplane, or just sit and breathe.

When there is more glucose in the body than can be used for energy, small amounts of the excess can be stored in the liver and muscles as glycogen, a starchy substance also referred to as "animal starch." But, for the most part, the carbohydrates eaten in excess of the body's energy needs are quickly converted to body fat. So you can become overweight by eating too many calories in carbohydrate form. But this is also true of excess protein calories and excess fat calories. Carbohydrates are no more "fattening" than the other two main nutrients. Excess calories in any form will add extra baggage for you to haul around. However, the rate each is metabolized may be different.

It is a common misconception that carbohydrates, especially the starches, are more fattening than other foods. In so thinking people have avoided breads, potatoes, and rice in an attempt to lose weight. A gram of carbohydrate yields four calories. A gram of protein yields the same. But for fats it is more than double: nine calories per gram. Ironically, if you reduce the quantity of carbohydrates in the diet, you usually eat more proteins, which are usually accompanied by fat. This produces the opposite of the desired results by actually increasing the total calorie intake. Calories do count! Approximately 3,500 extra calories result in a pound. It's not complicated—just simple arithmetic. It's essentially fuel management.

The major carbohydrate sources are grains (corn, rice, wheat, oats), products made from grains (flour, bread, breakfast cereal, spaghetti, noodles, macaroni, grits), potatoes, dried beans and peas, tapioca, sugar beets, and sugar cane. Most fruits and vegetables have smaller amounts of carbohydrates. In vegetables carbohydrates are chiefly in the starch form. In fruits they are mainly in the sugar.

Carbohydrates on the whole are very economical to produce in large quantities—a fact that the majority of the people in the world depend on for survival. Many countries rely on bread, potatoes, or rice to sustain their populations. Americans draw about half their total calories from carbohydrates, but of these, too many calories are consumed as white table sugar, soft drinks, cakes, candy, and processed food. Americans eat too many empty calories in forms that are deficient in vitamins and minerals and have detrimental side effects.

Sugar is used to flavor many foods and to provide quick energy. But foods high in sugar (sucrose) are high in calories and low in nutrient content. Refined sugar is an atypical food because it is pure carbohydrate—or pure calories. It has no protein, fat, vitamins, or minerals. Most other foods contain combinations of valuable nutrients, but not sugar. It is empty. What's worse, these empty calories tend to dull the appetite, further decreasing the intake of the valuable nutrients.

Sugars should only be eaten in moderation, but in the United States sugar consumption has been abused, and the level has reached about 100 pounds per person per year! This is because Americans are eating more concentrated sources of sugar as sweet manufactured products: soft drinks, bakery goods, cakes and candy, syrups, jams, and jellies. This all contributes to the high incidence of obesity and diabetes in the United States.

Many fresh fruits, raw and cooked vegetables, and whole grain cereals supply us with what we call bulk or roughage. The more popular term today is *fiber*. Fiber is the stiff, woody part of plants that supports, coats, or protects plant cells. It is composed of complex carbohydrates such as cellulose. For the most part, fiber is undigested as it goes through the digestive system, but it has some beneficial effects on the way. As the unused food mass passes through the intestines, fiber helps to make the stool softer and bulkier to speed passage and aid regularity. Fiber also may increase the elimination of bile acids, sterols, and fats. Scientists are studying other possible benefits of fiber in relation to disease prevention. One possible benefit is in preventing cancer of the colon.

FATS

Fats have a variety of functions. As one of the three basic components of our food, fat is a very concentrated source of energy which can be used for all types of work and body processes. Gram for gram, fat yields more than twice as much energy when metabolized than either protein or carbohydrates. And if those extra calories are not used for energy, then they will be applied to fat deposits or adipose tissue found just beneath the skin. Once again, the rule applies that excess calories put unwanted pounds on the body no matter the source.

Some fat deposits are beneficial. A certain amount of fat in the tissues helps to cushion the vital organs for added protection against traumatic injury. Some fat deposits in the body serve as a sort of insulation to aid in maintaining proper body temperature. However, too much fat deposited in the body not only makes you overweight and unbecoming but also disrupts all other body functions and can lead to serious, complicated health problems.

Supplying energy is the primary function of fat, and in this way it helps the body use protein and carbohydrates more efficiently for other purposes. But there are several other functions, too. Fats carry the fat-soluble vitamins A, D, E, and K, which are an essential part of any diet. Fats also aid in the actual absorption of these vitamins. Fats add flavor and variety of texture to many of our foods. They can give you a satisfied feeling because they are digested slowly and delay the stimulation of a hunger sensation. Certain fats must be included in the diet to provide the body with linoleic acid, an essential fatty acid that the body cannot synthesize on its own. Linoleic acid is indispensable for life. It is necessary for growth, reproduction, and healthy skin. You can find it especially in vegetable oils like corn, cottonseed, safflower, sesame, soybean, and wheat germ. It is also found in some nuts, poultry, and fish.

The most common fats found in our food are known as triglycerides. As the name implies, they are chemically composed of three fatty acids plus one glycerol, which is an alcohol. As dietary fats are digested, they are broken down into fatty acids and glycerol, the smaller building blocks. They are used by the body in this simpler form.

Nutritionists classify fatty acids in three categories: saturated, monounsaturated, and polyunsaturated, as TV commercials affirm. The names may sound complicated, but their meanings are simple. Each fatty acid is composed of carbon atoms joined like a chain, with as many as twenty carbons linked together. Every carbon atom has as many hydrogen atoms attached to it as it can hold. Like a sponge that is saturated with water and cannot absorb another drop, a saturated fatty acid contains the maximum number of hydrogens that it can hold. The unsaturated fatty acids, whether mono- or poly-, have some hydrogens missing from the molecule. A monounsaturated fatty acid has one location where hydrogen is missing and carbons have double-bonded to each other instead. A polyunsaturated has two or more locations where hydrogens are missing in the same fashion. These terms simply refer to the chemical structure of the molecules. But you have heard them used more often in reference to their physical and dietary differences.

One of the differences between saturated and unsaturated fatty acids is in their physical properties. Saturated fats are usually solid at room temperature and are composed of longer carbon chains. Unsaturated fats are usually liquid at room temperature and are composed of shorter chains. Although all of the fats, whether from plant or animal sources, are composed of a combination of both saturated and unsaturated fatty acids, the fats from animal sources such as butter, lard, or bacon generally are more saturated and solid at room temperature than the vegetable sources, like the liquid polyunsaturated vegetable oils. Of course, there are exceptions and variations within each group. For instance, in the meat group, beef and pork are much higher in saturated fats than poultry and fish, even though they all are from animal sources. The degree of saturation also may be altered in some cases, like in margarine. Vegetable oils are hydrogenated (they have hydrogens added to them) to make them more saturated and more solid, resulting in margarine.

It's important to understand the extent of saturation or unsaturation of foods because of the influence of saturation on the body's use of cholesterol. Cholesterol is a fatlike substance found naturally in the body. It is a normal ingredient in the blood and is found in every cell. Some of the cholesterol is made by the body, and some comes from food. Cholesterol is only found in foods of animal origin and is not present in plants (fruits, vegetables, grains, legumes, nuts, or vegetable oils). The amount of cholesterol included in the diet is one factor that affects the level of cholesterol in the bloodstream. It is generally accepted that saturated fats tend to increase the cholesterol level in the blood, polyunsaturates decrease blood cholesterol, and monounsaturates have no significant effect either way. Therefore, go for the polyunsaturates (vegetable source) and ease up on the saturates (animal source).

Researchers have concluded that the presence of high blood cholesterol contributes to atherosclerosis disease in many people. Atherosclerosis is a progressive, deteriorating process where fatty substances flowing in the bloodstream are deposited on the inner walls of the arteries. In time the deposit enlarges to inhibit the flow of blood, and it eventually may block an entire artery. This diminishes or ends the supply of nutrients and oxygen to the particular tissue that this artery feeds, and the tissue is impaired or dies. When an artery in the brain is blocked, some of the brain tissue dies, and the result is a stroke. When an artery in the heart itself, a coronary artery, becomes blocked, part of the heart tissue dies and becomes ineffective, resulting in a heart attack. Either can be fatal or, at best, disabling. So consider cholesterol to be one item in a group of risk factors that leads to heart disease. This does not mean that you should radically change your diet, for there are no guarantees, but you should moderate total fat consumption in addition to trying to lower high blood pressure, stop smoking, lose excessive weight, and increase exercise.

WATER AND HYDRATION

Water is a nutrient essential for life. You can live without food for days or even up to two weeks, but you can only last a few days without water.

About two-thirds of body weight is water. Water serves as a building material, a solvent for all products of digestion, the medium of body fluids (secretions and excretions), a regulator of body temperature by means of evaporation through skin and lungs, a carrier of nutrients and waste products from one part of the body to another, an aid in digestion, and a necessary part in all chemical reactions of metabolism.

The right amount of water is maintained in the body by a part of the brain controlling thirst. When your body is running low on water, you feel thirsty; you are dehydrated. Unfortunately, the sense of thirst does not happen until after you become dehydrated. Dehydration leads to fatigue and poor flying performance. When there is too much water, it is excreted by the kidneys in urine. You cannot drink too much water, especially while flying.

Water losses need to be replaced in the body every day in generous amounts. Water usually is supplied by drinking, but there also is water in foods. There is no magic number of glasses of water that you should consume every day (though six to eight is usually recommended). Instead, let nature be your guide.

VITAMINS

In terms of quantity or mass, our foods consist mostly of protein, carbohydrates, fats, and water. These substances are essential for building a healthy body but would be useless without vitamins and minerals, which are smaller in quantity and not as visible.

Vitamins are quite popular in the health scene today. Many people are aware of the importance of vitamins. There are controversies, however, as to what amount of each vitamin should be included in the diet. It is important that we get the right amounts because either too little or too much of a vitamin can cause serious illnesses. We use vitamins in extremely minute amounts, milligrams and micrograms, so even a small excess amount of certain vitamins can be toxic. It is erroneous to assume with vitamins that "if a little of something is good, then a lot is better." But still, the per capita consumption of vitamins is steadily increasing in the pill-popping United States.

Vitamins have dynamic functions in body processes, regulating many chemical reactions. They are essential for the release of energy from food, for normal growth of different tissues of the body, for controlling the body's use of food, and for proper functioning of nerves and muscles. They do not provide energy or build tissues. They have no calories. About fourteen major vitamins have been identified (there may be more) that are necessary for health. Recommended amounts have been established for ten of them. Each vitamin has a special function in the body, and no other nutrient can take its place or do its job. You must eat a variety of foods to consume a variety of vitamins.

Vitamins can be categorized into two classes, depending on whether they are soluble in fat or soluble in water. The water-soluble vitamins—C, thiamin, niacin, and riboflavin—mix in water as a solution. They are not stored by the body. Excesses of the water-soluble vitamins are excreted in the urine. Large doses of these vitamins create very expensive urine! The fat-soluble vitamins—A, D, E and K—are stored by the body and are not flushed out in the urine. They are not soluble in water, so care must be taken when consuming these because too much A, D, E or K in the body can be toxic.

Are you consuming enough vitamins? Should you be taking some vitamin supplements? Are you overdosing on any vitamins already? The answers to these questions are not simple. Obviously, it is impossible for you to know exactly what is taking place inside your own cells down to the microgram level. But a tremendous amount of research has been conducted to establish some guidelines for eating and some requirements for daily intake of vitamins. The investigations continue, and modifications are being made in the guidelines as more evidence is revealed. In the meantime you need to be wise about your eating practices. A pattern of three or more small, regular meals each day, of a well-chosen variety of foods, taken in moderation should provide you with adequate amounts of vitamins.

If you have some way of knowing that you are not getting all of the nutrients that you need (if you are not eating right, if you are skipping meals, if you are not eating an assortment of fruits, vegetables, meats, milk, and grains, or if you are replacing too many real foods with junk foods), then you need a conservative multivitamin supplement—not necessarily a megavitamin. Again, use moderation.

Vitamins are indispensable and play a vital role in keeping us healthy by assisting in numerous processes of growth and development. They inhibit diseases such as scurvy, beriberi, anemia, and rickets. Lately, the vitamin industry is profiting from misleading claims that certain vitamins provide endless energy and physical endurance, a better sex life, instant relief from colds, guaranteed good health, slowing of the aging process, elimination of body odor, and prevention of gray hair. Vitamins do contribute to feeling great, but be leery of exaggerations and single incidents that are not yet supported by scientific evidence. Also, be aware that, as a result of frivolous, superficial advertising and a rather careless public attitude, vitamins have developed the connotation of being harmless candy. Actually vitamins are chemicals with very complex molecular structures and long chemical names. Eating excessive amounts of vitamins may have adverse side effects. Some of the symptoms of hypervitaminosis are fatigue, weight loss, pains, skin changes, loss of appetite, changes in elimination, abdominal discomfort, insomnia, high blood pressure, headaches, nausea, and vomiting. Massive doses of certain vitamins can cause death. So vitamins should be taken as carefully as any drug.

MINERALS

About 4 to 5 percent of your total body weight is made up of minerals, another group of nutrients essential for living. They are natural elements that have important contributions to make to vital body functions. Over fifteen are known to be required, and daily recommended allowances have been established for six of them. Like vitamins, minerals do not provide calories, so they do not supply energy. They are not broken down in the body but are absorbed from the digestive tract in the same form as they occur in foods. Minerals are not used up by the body; instead, they enter, carry out their specific functions, and are excreted. (Iron is the exception. It is stored and reused.) This is why minerals must be replaced regularly by eating a balanced, varied diet. If you are not eating adequate meals, consider taking a moderate daily supplement. Some of the most prominent minerals are calcium, phosphorus, iodine, and iron.

Calcium is the most abundant mineral in the body, making up about two to three pounds. Almost all of it is concentrated in the bones and teeth, giving them strength and rigidity. The small amount of calcium in the rest of the body tissues and fluids aids in the clotting of the blood, contraction of muscles, transmission of nerve impulses, heart functions, regulation of fluids, and activation of enzymes. Calcium deficiency results in rickets (in children) and osteoporosis, the softening of bones. Calcium is found especially in milk and cheeses.

Phosphorus also is a main ingredient for building bones and teeth. It also helps regulate energy within the body cells. It is easily obtained; good sources are meat, poultry, fish, eggs, and whole-grain foods.

Iodine is vital to the normal function of the thyroid gland, which controls metabolism. It is required in extremely small amounts, but getting too little can cause goiter, a swelling of the thyroid gland. People who live inland where the soil contains little iodine sometimes fail to get adequate amounts. Iodized table salt and seafood are good sources of iodine.

Iron is needed in small but important amounts. It combines with protein to make hemoglobin, the red substance of blood that carries oxygen to the cells and carbon dioxide to the lungs to be exhaled. Too little iron in the diet or chronic blood loss can cause iron deficiency anemia. Liver is an excellent source of iron. Other sources are organ meats, shellfish, lean meats, egg yolks, dark green leafy vegetables, dried fruit, molasses, and whole-grain cereals.

Other minerals include chlorine, cobalt, copper, fluorine, magnesium, potassium, manganese, sodium, sulfur, zinc, chromium, selenium, and molybdenum.

THE CHECKLIST

Checklists, checklists, checklists—as a pilot you are more than familiar with the idea of using a checklist. A checklist is a record of things to do in a certain order. It serves as a tool in accomplishing a specific task, whether that be a preflight or an emergency procedure. The purpose of each checklist is to make the task easier, faster, and safer to accomplish and more accurate. It ensures that no items are missed. Following a systematic checklist simplifies the pilot's job, saves valuable time in situations where seconds count, and limits the possibility of human error.

In a similar fashion, when it comes to eating properly, there are special checklists, too. By faithfully following these eating checklists you can be assured that you are getting all of the nutrients that you need each day. They are quite accurate and very simple to use.

Why bother? Well, considering the three basic nutrients—protein, carbohydrates, and fat—plus all of the different vitamins and minerals, you've got about forty to fifty total nutrients to keep track of. If you had nothing better to do, you could befriend a computer and spend all of your waking hours doing scientific research to determine your individual nutrient needs and how much of this and that to eat. But, as you most likely would rather spend your time flying, you're in luck: nutrition scientists have done the hard part already. Information has been reduced to lists of recommended daily allowances (RDA) of each nutrient for certain ages and energy needs. They are intended to be guidelines for all healthy people and are generous enough to accommodate the individual variations among the normal population living in the United States who are under normal amounts of environmental stress. They serve as a guide for planning food intake.

This daily food checklist arranges foods into four groups according to content, because certain types of food have common nutrients occurring in approximately the same quantity. Each food usually contains more than one type of nutrient, but no single food supplies all forty to fifty nutrients. So it is important to eat a variety of foods in moderation. Based on the amounts of each nutrient needed daily for proper growth, maintenance, and repair, scientists were able to recommend the amount of foods to eat in terms of number of servings from each of four general food groups. In case you think it is too simple or too old-fashioned, remember that this is not based on a fad. According to the RDA, you can choose from an endless assortment of food to suit your taste, family budget, caloric need, stage of life, and need for weight control. The food group pattern for a healthy diet is the same as it has been for many years, but we have learned better how to adjust for individual needs within the guidelines.

Keep in mind two very important concepts as you plan your meals: *variation* and *moderation.*

THERMODYNAMICS FOR AERODYNAMICS

Nutrition, as well as aeronautics, engineering, chemistry, physics, ecology, and every other discipline, is subject to laws of nature—laws that exist as an intrinsic part of creation and are not contrived by any of our own machinations. They are inescapable.

You are currently flying an incredible piece of equipment, but even that machine has limitations. Powerful as it is, it still must submit to the laws of nature. Each aircraft has its own particular maximum takeoff weight and maximum landing weight, for instance. These numerical values impose the upper limit of safety for the particular aerodynamics of that structure. It would be dangerous to ignore such limitations and to attempt to operate the aircraft beyond its capabilities; even someone who loves to push the envelope knows a max-grossed 747 can't be put into a vertical climb.

So what about you, the pilot of the aircraft? Consider your limits governed by the laws of nature. Each cell of your body is far more intricate than the aircraft. You contain infinitely complex chemical reactions that miraculously continue in spite of your abuse. Your heart labors unceasingly to sustain your life. What are its limits? When you took off this morning to start your day were you at your ideal weight or were you carrying ten or twenty pounds of extra baggage? Were you maintaining an airworthy anatomy? Are you putting undue stress on your heart muscle? If you tax your heart beyond its natural limits, something will give.

When an airplane is overgrossed with fuel beyond the maximum landing weight, there are two alternatives: burn it or dump it. You can continue in flight and burn fuel at the normal rate of consumption. A faster method is to dump fuel—to simply drop the excess from the plane. When you are overgrossed, wouldn't it be wonderful to be able to simply dump the excess baggage from your body? Fortunately and unfortunately, the human body doesn't work that way. The body is actually a more efficient machine than the aircraft. As a means of self-preservation, the body clutches any excess food fuel, stores it as fat, and saves it for a possible time when fuel may be scarce. But for many of us our storehouses are full to overflowing, and we experience few hard times. To lighten the load for the overworked heart, the extra fat must be burned off.

Each of us is a self-contained system of matter and energy, and like every other organism we are subject to some inescapable laws of nature governing development, growth, and change. Our physical equilibrium, or health, depends on these unchanging natural laws for the complex chemical reactions of matter and the conservation of energy (heat) within the system, the body. We cannot defy the laws of chemodynamics and thermodynamics that rule the human machine. But we can use these scientific properties to our advantage.

To maintain good health and an ideal weight you need to know your system and the laws that govern it. Don't be swayed by pushers of magical foods and hocus-pocus diets who claim to circumvent the natural processes and promise immediate results. You need to know the principles of matter and energy as they relate to the functions of eating and exercise. There is very little value to the temporary, two-week diet. Instead, develop a sensible eating style for life.

Energy from food is measured in units, or calories (technically kilocalories). All foods supply calories, but some supply many more than others. Calories are not nutrients; rather they are the amount of potential energy for bodily use that can be released from nutrients. (Getting really scientific, a calorie is the amount of heat needed to raise the temperature of one pint of water by four degrees Fahrenheit.)

The daily amount of calories you need depends mostly on your particular body size and your level of physical activity—or inactivity. Some other influencing factors are your age, sex, and stage of growth. At rest your body requires about one calorie per minute just to stay alive. This is like idling your engine. The motor is running, but you're not going anywhere. Some people exist this way—barely functioning and avoiding any extra exertion. The problem is that they may eat as much as others who are active.

Eating fats, carbohydrates, and proteins supplies the raw materials for growth and energy production when you need it. But eating an overabundance of them doesn't make you more energetic. In fact, eating more than you need causes storage of these materials in the form of adipose tissue. In plain terms the excess makes you fat and sluggish, not more active.

Excess calories may be hazardous to your health. Whether from fats, proteins, or carbohydrates, a calorie is a calorie is a calorie, no matter where it came from, and 3,500 unused calories make one pound of body fat. The accumulation of the 3,500 unburned calories may be sudden, as during the holiday season when people excuse themselves from restraints, or it may be gradual—a few calories here and a few more there and soon a pound sneaks up on you. Consider this situation: every day for one year you eat 100 calories in excess of what you need—just 100 calories each day beyond the point where you should have stopped. These may even be in the form of a nutritious food. One hundred excess calories each day may look like this:

1st day—a medium apple
2d day—a cookie
3d day—eight potato chips
4th day—two-thirds cup milk
5th day—one tablespoon butter
6th day—one slice of lunch meat
(getting the idea?)
363d day—one orange
364th day—one tablespoon salad dressing
365th day—one tablespoon cream in your coffee

The list looks pretty harmless, doesn't it? And a lot of the items are even good for you. But, 100 extra calories each day, whether from a nutritious apple or a cookie, for one year adds ten pounds of excess fat.

You can easily see that if this process is allowed to continue you can become obese. However, when the number of calories that you eat is equal to the calories that you use, your weight will remain stable, and when the number you consume is fewer than the number used, you will lose weight. Everyone has his or her own rate of metabolism, and recent studies suggest some people may have genes that make burning calories more easy or difficult. Still, maintaining a healthy weight depends on fuel management.

There are no magic foods or diets that flush fat out of the body. Weight gain, loss, or stability is a simple matter of addition and subtraction. The way to lose weight is to burn more calories than you eat or eat less than you burn, in other words, exercise more and eat less. Any eating/activity pattern (I avoid using the word *diet* because it implies something temporary) that creates a deficit in calories will cause you to lose weight. But since our goal is to stay slim and healthy, not merely slim, be sure that the foods that you do eat are the nutritious ones. While you are counting calories, you might as well throw out the foods that are purely empty calories, such as soda pop and sweets. Emphasize foods that are packed with vitamins and minerals.

Most people are at their ideal weight sometime between the age of twenty and twenty-five. After that, fewer and fewer calories are needed to keep the ideal weight, but people usually continue to eat the same amounts anyway just out of habit. Also, in later years they become less physically active, which further contributes pounds.

Prevention is the name of the game when it comes to your health. By periodically and routinely checking your bodily gauges and indicators for potential health risks, you may save your life. A thorough "physical preflight" can identify a possible problem in its early stages, in time for you to reduce the risk and thereby increase your years of good health and life expectancy. You have some built-in early warning systems if you will just stop and notice them.

Develop a risk factor consciousness for an effective physical. Risk factors are those characteristics of your medical history, family history, and medical status that are linked with high rates of premature death and disability from certain diseases. Risk is a statistical expression of probability of a greater likelihood of disease. The pertinent risk factors are such things as a high level of blood cholesterol, smoking, high blood pressure, diabetes, obesity, inappropriate diet, stress, age, gender, lack of exercise, an abnormal electrocardiogram, and heredity.

Some of your risk factors can be modified or even removed. In so doing, you can improve your health and maybe increase your overall life expectancy. You can't do anything about your gender, heredity, and age, but you can work on the other risk factors. Losing excess weight reduces the risk of heart disease and stroke, helps to prevent or delay diabetes, lowers blood pressure, and lowers blood fat and buildup of atherosclerosis.

IN REVIEW

Incorporating healthy eating habits and proper physical activity into your lifestyle can greatly enhance and probably extend your productive years. Health maintenance may also prevent your being grounded by the FAA for a disorder caused by diet and inactivity.

Whether shopping for groceries, preparing a meal, eating at home, enjoying a dinner party, sneaking a snack, ordering in a restaurant, consuming a crew meal, potlucking at a picnic, or raiding the refrigerator, the same philosophy in making food choices should prevail. Use wisdom to develop a prudent eating style. Here are some tips:

- Eat a wide variety of foods from each of the four food groups.
- Eat moderate amounts. Purposefully eat only half of what is on your plate at each meal. Overeating is hazardous to your health.
- Emphasize consuming foods in their original state: fresh fruit, fresh vegetables, and whole grains.

- Deemphasize consuming animal products (beef, pork, butter, and eggs) and heavily processed foods.
- Beware of table salt and white sugar. Also watch out for sodium and sugars hidden in processed foods.
- Eliminate the "unfoods" with the empty calories like pop, candy, and pastries.
- Read nutrition labels for calorie content and nutrient breakdown. Ingredient lists are usually arranged in order of decreasing amounts. If a sugar, sodium, nitrites, or other villains are listed early in the list, select a different item.
- Eat slowly. Take more time to enjoy the flavor and texture of each food. Try new foods.

If you are trying to lose weight, you must eat nutritional foods and burn more calories than you eat or eat fewer than you burn. Shedding fat is possible, but there is no immediate, safe, magical way. Avoid the extremes of fad reducing diets and gimmicks. They may appear to be effective temporarily but in the long run can be harmful to your health. A change in your long-range eating style is best. Eating a wide variety of foods in moderation is your best bet. Remember that 3,500 calories make one pound, so cut back on calories in meals and snacks. Here are some more tips:

- Since calories count, count them! Try keeping a food diary for several days, listing foods eaten, portion sizes, and number of calories. It will be an eye-opener. You will be able to identify problem foods in your diet and eliminate them. It's not as boring as it sounds. Many pilots have done this.
- Snacks, beverages, and "tastes" have calories, too.
- Diet pills do not work. In addition, they can raise your blood pressure to unacceptable levels.
- Limit fats, refined sugar, and alcoholic beverages.
- Work with someone who has the same goals. It's amazing how much more diligent we are when held accountable by someone else.
- Prepare your plate with care. Don't surround yourself with bowls of food at the table that tease you into taking seconds. You don't have to eat everything on your plate.
- Exercise. Physical activity is a great help. It burns calories and curbs the appetite.
- Put a copy of your medical certificate on your refrigerator door as a reminder of how important your health is.

8

An Exercise Program for Pilots

A thirty-five-year-old airline pilot was noted to have a variation in his ECG, and because the ECG was the first one submitted to the FAA, he was asked by the FAA for more evaluation. The pilot was out of shape, had a high resting pulse rate, and was a heavy coffee drinker. His obviously poor condition was cured by an exercise program, and he stopped drinking excessive amounts of coffee. His ECG returned to normal. However, the additional evaluation, which turned out to be OK, also had to be reported to the FAA.

In the 1970s there was an increased interest by Americans in physical fitness. No longer was the lone jogger someone to stare at. This was not a passing fad: as more people became more active and realized the benefits, others took notice and began their own exercise programs. Such programs have passed the test of time and, in the majority of cases, have withstood criticism. The concept of health maintenance is alive and well and has become a big business.

In early 1995, medical specialists agreed that a sedentary lifestyle was an independent risk factor for the development of heart disease. This means that, by itself (not in combination with other factors such as elevated cholesterol and blood pressure), not exercising means you have a higher chance of experiencing heart problems. The way to reduce that risk is to add physical activity in any form to your lifestyle.

However, if an exercise program truly prolongs life and maintains good health and a sense of well-being, why aren't all pilots, especially professional pilots, participating in some sort of exercise program? Certainly beginning and continuing an exercise program is not a simple task, but with a career at stake, why the apathy?

Let's begin by defining why exercise is important both physiologically and psychologically. Unlike other machines, the performance and efficiency of the human machine improves if it is worked under controlled conditions. This leads to a quality of health that all of us envy. What then are the special qualities that result from an active exercise program? And what does the term *exercise* really mean?

First, those who exercise improve the efficiency of their lungs. They are better able to use the oxygen that they inhale and to exhale impurities and carbon dioxide. Those who exercise realize that they no longer have to huff and puff for usual, mildly strenuous activities such as going up and down stairs. Their capacity for work increases, and the necessity to breathe harder when working decreases. They finally can keep up with their children instead of blaming their need to slow down on age. And while taking a brisk walk with a friend, they can carry on an active conversation without frequently pausing to catch their breath.

Equally important is the improvement of heart muscle efficiency. The heart muscle is like other muscles in the body that weaken and become flabby without strenuous use. Granted, the heart is pumping all the time but only in a mild way, especially if we lead a sedentary life. The way to exercise the heart muscle is to make it work harder over a prolonged period. Those who participate in an exercise program notice that they can tolerate the stress of hard work and prolonged exercise with much greater ease without a pounding heart, shortness of breath, and racing pulse. They also notice that their *resting* pulse is lower than it used to be. That is, instead of being at 88 in a resting situation, it is now in the 60s. Obviously, that lower pulse rate is an indication that the heart muscle is far more efficient than it used to be and needs to beat less frequently; it has a far more efficient hydraulic pressure and subsequent movement of blood with each beat.

An unexpected, but pleasant, spin-off of a physical-conditioning program is a general feeling of well-being. The entire body feels better, fatigues less easily, and seems to have more energy. The body is also far more resistant to diseases and other complications that result from the abuses it is subjected to in daily life.

Contrary to popular opinion, an exercise program is not the sole method for weight loss, although it is an essential part of any program. You cannot run a mile and then gorge yourself with all the food that you know you shouldn't be eating and then expect to lose weight. Remember, one pound of fat is equal to about 3,500 calories. You can either walk, run, or jog one mile, but you will use only 100 calories in the process—the human machine is extremely efficient in its use of calories. In order to burn off the pound of fat you have stored and accumulated by overeating, you would have to run thirty-five miles! That is a pretty high price to pay for overindulgence.

Exercise does use up calories, though, and certainly over time it is a great companion to a weight-reduction program. For example, if you were to walk an extra mile a day, that's 100 more calories burned. If you also eat 100 calories less a day, that's a total of 200 calories, and over a month's period, that's about 6,000 calories, or about two pounds of weight loss. It requires discipline, but if you are willing to wait for results, the combination is rewarding and lasting.

There is increasing evidence that, in addition to burning additional calories, exercise enhances the metabolic process of losing weight. Exercise and counting calories are synergistic.

So how can you tell if you are improving your physical condition from a good program? What are the tangible and objective results that you can see? Probably the most important guide is your pulse rate. We should all be familiar with our resting pulse rate. (It should be no more than 75–85 and ideally in the low to mid 60s.) With moderate exercise, your pulse shouldn't go much above 150, and it should return to normal or slightly above a resting rate after a minimal amount of rest (ten to twenty minutes). These guides are an indication that the heart is working efficiently and is in good physical condition. Get in the habit of frequently checking your pulse.

Your blood pressure, if elevated, will also begin to come down with exercise, but not as noticeably as your pulse rate. You might notice an increased ability to tolerate the stresses of life, whether they be psychological or physical. You might also notice that you have more energy and are able to enjoy activity after returning home from a long trip. Your endurance should increase.

You will feel and look good. People will begin to notice that you are a different person, and you will begin to realize that the way you used to feel was certainly not worth the overindulgence in food, cigarettes, or alcohol. You will find yourself suffering from fewer colds and flus, and if you do have an illness, you will bounce back more quickly. Obviously, no one can guarantee total absence of illness, but certainly you can return to flying much sooner than someone whose sedentary lifestyle has resulted in poor physical condition.

In early 1995, medical specialists agreed that there was another independent risk factor for the development of heart disease—a sedentary lifestyle. This means that by itself, and not in combination with other factors such as elevated cholesterol and blood pressure, not exercising gives you a higher chance of having heart problems.

Non–insulin-dependent diabetes (type II) is often controlled with a good diet and exercise program. Studies have shown that type II diabetes can actually be prevented with good exercise. If you have a family history of diabetes and feel you are at risk, an exercise program is essential.

With so many good reasons to exercise, let's examine for a moment why so many of us do not. The biggest obstacle is laziness, which, interestingly, is a result of not exercising. Therefore, it results in a vicious circle. In addition, we expect immediate results. Once we are turned on to an exercise program, if we don't see results in a few days, we become discouraged and slip back into our old habits, especially if the program bores you. Pilots are used to seeing the effects of their efforts within minutes or hours. This certainly is not true in an exercise program. Therefore, we rationalize and find excuses such as "exercising is too boring," "I never have enough time," "it's too lonely," "I don't know where to exercise," and "I would rather spend the time with my family." You and I have heard all of these before, and I am sure that each of you has also expressed them. Until you have actually experienced the feelings of being in good physical condition, an exercise program won't likely become a top priority. Interestingly, those who do find time to exercise tend to be more efficient in the use of their time and accomplish far more than those who do not.

Unfortunately, one of the greatest incentives to begin an exercise program is when AMEs tell pilots that their blood pressure is too high and that they are grounded until they lower it. One can imagine the efforts that the pilots make to exercise. The pilots will realize what they have been missing and will continue to participate in this physical conditioning since they do not want to feel the way they used to. They will become proud of the way they look and the fact that they are able to endure conditions they weren't able to tolerate in the past.

But being grounded is a poor way to get your attention. A better way is to commit yourself to another person, be it your spouse, a friend, or someone else who has the same difficulty in following a program. However, you must accept the fact that you need to exercise before you can subject yourself to the eventual problems you will face starting and continuing the program. Until you begin to notice the benefits, the job will be tough. With irregular hours, overnight stays in various locations, and fatigue from long trips, you have actual deterrents to following a program. However, you do have options that will accommodate your schedule.

You probably know a number of people who have been able to resolve similar difficulties and are now following a commendable physical conditioning program. These are the people you should talk with. Allow them to share their methods and ways of overcoming the deterrents. Once you have faced the issue of needing to start a program, and have found someone to share the program with, you must choose a type of exercise and schedule it so it will be productive for you. You will probably have to develop two programs: one that you can practice at home and one you can do on trips.

Many people think that an exercise program is limited to jogging. Jogging turns some people off, and if that's your feeling, then jogging is not what you should be doing. Jogging is also hard on the body, and there are studies that indicate that, for some people, more damage is caused than benefit achieved, especially long-term. There are many alternatives. Admittedly, jogging may produce results more quickly than other forms of exercise. A brisk walk can result in the same aerobic benefits, but it does take a greater time commitment.

All the respected books on exercise programs basically have one goal, and that is what we will discuss now. One word of caution: even a little exercise is better than nothing, provided that it is not the type where you exert yourself beyond your capacities during a short period once a week. It is better to commit yourself to a few minutes a day and then to build up to a more complete program than to try to make up for lost time on the weekends. The weekend athlete is a prime target for sudden medical disorders such as sore backs, sprained ankles, and even heart attacks. The other extreme is someone who gets so turned on by an exercise program that he or she becomes extremely competitive and starts running seven, eight, or even nine miles a day or playing aggressive handball to the point where this person is risking injury.

The secret to any good exercise program is simply this: after a ten-minute warm-up of stretching, walking, calisthenics, walking in place, or so on, progress into exercise that raises your pulse to the target rate specific for your age and keep it there for about twenty minutes. A common formula to establish your target rate is to subtract your age from 240—that's your maximum target rate for the exercise portion. If you can achieve 80 percent or more of that rate, you are in an effective program.

Then gradually cool down for another ten minutes by either slowing the activities or going back to the calisthenics, slow walking, or stretching. At no time should you jump into vigorous exercise and then suddenly stop and go about your usual business. A warm-up, cool-down, and stretching program is essential. There are some studies that indicate that stretching is not necessary, but it still seems prudent to include some when warming up.

Forty to sixty minutes two to three times a week certainly is not much of a sacrifice of time, but it is amazing how often we can rationalize allegedly better uses for those few moments. Another part of the secret to success is that you should not allow more than two or three days to elapse between exercise sessions.

Pulse is an indicator of how you are doing. Keep a written record of your pulse. Know what your resting pulse is, how long it takes you to get up to your target rate, and how long it takes you to get down to your resting pulse after exercise. Techniques for determining what these rates should be and how they can be improved are more fully explained in the many books on exercise programs. An incentive you might use is to keep a chart with resting, exercising, and cool-down pulses. Post it where everybody can see it; that way you can't cheat. You might put a copy of your medical certificate above this graph to remind you of why you're going to the trouble. Placing the certificate next to a diet and weight chart also is a strong motivator. You can even begin to compete with a member of your family or a friend so you can keep track of each other's progress and give and get support to continue.

The type of exercise best for you is probably the hardest thing to determine. Again, books and quick to read manuals very nicely explain the alternatives and how they relate to each other in terms of output and efficiency. In addition to jogging, running, and walking, don't forget about jumping rope, small minitrampolines that can be used in the house, stationary bikes, treadmills, and competitive sports. Equipment like treadmills and stationary cross country ski tracks have been very popular. Structured aerobic exercises demonstrated on videotapes and in sports clubs are effective. Many of these programs you can do at home, but they may be somewhat more difficult for you to pursue when you are on a trip. If you check into a motel where you can either swim, go up and down several flights of stairs, jump rope, or just go for a long walk, you've found an ideal place to stay. Certainly with your health and career at stake, it would behoove you to find places where your exercise program can be followed. It is my understanding that an increasing number of hotels and motels are providing access to exercise facilities, especially if they cater to flight crews.

The main point here is that you should experiment with different kinds of exercise. If you don't like one, try another. But don't give up on an exercise program simply because you can't find one you like.

IN REVIEW

I recommend reading a few books that will give you alternative ways to achieve the goal of increasing your pulse over a gradual period of time, keeping it there for a minimum of twenty minutes, and then cooling down. Even if you are not sure how you are going to like it, at least go out and buy the jump rope or jogging shoes or treadmill. Commit yourself to at least three or four weeks before you decide that you can't or don't want to pursue a specific program, and then try another. Find out how others overcame their hang-ups. Most important of all, do something, share it with somebody else, and keep an ongoing record.

9
Habits and Abuses That Affect Your Certification, and Miscellaneous Medical Topics

Each of the habits discussed in this chapter can be controlled by self-commitment and self-control. We all can identify with these habits; we see them in ourselves and in our flying comrades, habits that some people abstain from and others overindulge in.

As a professional pilot, you picked a career in which you must maintain your health. Each one of the subjects discussed in this chapter can affect that vital medical certificate. Those who have more than one bad habit have a greater probability of a disappointing future. Perhaps when you reach for a cigarette or that extra cup of coffee or that last "one for the road," you'll remember some of the comments made in this book.

SMOKING

Everyone knows that smoking is a major risk factor in developing heart disease and pulmonary complications. Nobody has been able to justify why he or she smokes other than the habit developed initially because of enjoyment and eventually became addictive because of nicotine. Smoking and other tobacco products, especially "smokeless tobacco," continue to be the sole source of nicotine, a very strong stimulant to the heart and blood vessels; a major cause of malignancies; and a source of carbon monoxide, which adds to your already hypoxic condition while flying.

If you wish you had a choice of which disease you could acquire, pick cancer because of its finality. Emphysema, a lung disorder directly related to smoking, is a horrible way to live because it is very difficult to breath under even the most minimal of exertions. Bronchitis is a continuing and progressive source of infection. Significant coronary artery disease is a mandatory disqualification for medical certification.

The carbon monoxide of a burning cigarette is a major factor leading to increased hypoxia, decreased night vision, and more noticeable fatigue, especially after a trip. Often those who smoke also consume vast amounts of caffeine, which means that the "let down," or withdrawal, from this overstimulated state prevents you from relaxing.

Equally important is the insult to those who do not like or cannot tolerate smoke. Not only are you insulting others you are subjecting them to the same medical abuses that you have chosen.

Most smokers want to stop. A few have succeeded, most have at least cut down (which is very important—cutting down decreases your health risks), but there are those who continue to be heavy smokers in spite of the facts. It seems apparent to me, as a doctor, that I cannot scare smokers; they are already aware of the consequences. I suggest to those who want to quit that they must first truly want to; if they don't, they might as well not even try. Their frustrations will be taken out not only on themselves but on those around them.

As with other bad habits, controlling your smoking cannot always be done alone. If you are willing to commit yourself to somebody else and establish your priorities with another person, he or she can be supportive and guide you during the more tempting moments. There are many support groups and techniques, and they may be worthwhile if they get the job done. But if you can't quit for yourself, at least do it for those who depend upon and care about you. It is difficult enough to put up with the stench of smoke on your breath, the tobacco and ash on your clothes, and the risk that you are facing. As a professional pilot, denying yourself and your family a career simply because you like cigarettes is a perfect example of someone who has the wrong priorities.

Smoking has become less of an issue for airlines, with few pilots still smoking and smoking forbidden in the cockpit and passenger cabin in most airlines and many corporate aircraft. Unfortunately, there remains a surprising number of people who have taken up or continue to use chewing tobacco, particularly young people, our next generation of pilots. These people absorb far more nicotine than they do from cigarettes, increase their chances of cancer in the mouth, and annoy others with chewing and spitting.

CAFFEINE

Coffee and tea are a part of our social lifestyle and certainly a part of the "after-takeoff checklist." The caffeine found in coffee, tea, most cola products, and some chocolates, however, is more than a simple stimulant to get us going in the morning. To some this caffeine is a very strong stimulant to the heart muscle and nervous system. In addition, it affects our minds in the sense that it makes us oversensitive, anxious, and in some cases neurotic. I have known cases of pilots who have been grounded because of an abnormality in their ECG that was purely a result of too much caffeine. They had some extra beats (PVCs, or premature ventricular contractions) and other rhythm problems directly related to this overstimulation. Caffeine also acts as a diuretic. That is, it promotes the formation and excretion of urine. For example, you can drink one cup of coffee and urinate three cups of water. In an already desert-dry flight deck, this easily leads to dehydration and fatigue. Caffeine can be very troublesome to some stomachs. While it may not necessarily cause ulcers, it is an overstimulant to the acid secretions. Some decaffeinated coffee is equally irritating.

The problem with caffeine is not the drug itself, but the amount that is consumed. You don't normally need that second cup of coffee, especially when you are flying or working. But drinking it becomes a habit, something to do with your hands, and you could just as easily drink coffee-flavored hot water. Overstimulation from caffeine and its dehydrating effect make you tense and fatigued not only during the trip but especially afterward. It prevents you from resting comfortably and relaxing. Therefore, the withdrawal effects after a trip are a form of impairment and certainly distracting at the very least, especially if you have another leg to fly in an hour or so. Recent studies confirm that caffeine is addictive, and if you regularly drink only one to two cups a day, you could suffer withdrawal if you try to quit suddenly, with symptoms including headaches, nervousness, and inability to sleep. It's better to cut back over a period of several days.

Controlling your caffeine intake is no different than controlling any other habit. You must first identify how much caffeine you are consuming and then find a substitute. In most cases, the first cup of coffee at the beginning of the trip is perfectly acceptable. After that, however, find substitutes, such as juices, highly diluted decaffeinated coffee, or noncola beverages. Certainly make a habit of drinking several cups of water between those other beverages. An important point to keep in mind is that every time you are offered a cup of coffee ask for something else, even if it's just a glass of water. I think you will find the results after the trip most satisfying.

ALCOHOL

You do not have to be an alcoholic to suffer the effects of even small amounts of alcohol in your system. Most of us who drink alcoholic beverages do so because of their flavor and euphoric effect and because they reduce our inhibitions. But, in addition, it is a strong stimulant to the cardiovascular system that makes us more excitable and makes the heart work harder—adrenaline seems to be higher. This is why you feel your heart pumping harder the day after a big party. The problem is that if you were to plot the euphoria from one highball, that effect lasts for a shorter time than the effects of the stimulant. Therefore, as you drink more, you actually add to the stimulant curve. The result is the euphoria disappears in a matter of hours, but the stimulant effect will be around for twelve to twenty-four hours. In addition, it prevents you from getting your REM sleep (the sleep necessary for your body to be completely rested). In this sense, alcohol seems to have the same effect as barbiturates, which also reduce REM sleep. You may pass out after a party, but you will not be rested by the next morning.

In addition, alcohol acts as a diuretic, causing dehydration. However, you can't simply drink water to recover. No one really knows what causes a hangover, but fluid imbalance plays a role. The fluid volume within your body increases (since the diuretic effect of alcohol lasts for only a short period of time), preventing you from losing more fluids. This added fluid in addition to the blood vessel expansion, especially in your head, is thought to lead to the miserable headache the day following excessive consumption.

As you drink more over time, you can tolerate more. On the other hand, if you haven't always been a heavy drinker, you tend to be more affected by smaller amounts as you age. Therefore how alcohol affects you will depend greatly upon the conditions under which you are drinking. The consequences of alcohol can affect you up to two days—the withdrawal effects, the stimulative effects, and the fatigue. The effect of alcohol on the stomach has led many an ulcer to bleed. Also, those who drink a lot often smoke a lot, and this combination can increase medical risks. Those who think drinking a lot of coffee the following morning will help are wrong. What they end up doing is compounding the overstimulated effects on the heart.

The next time you experience the "morning after the night before," consider how what you are feeling—the pounding heart, the headache, the dehydration, and the fatigue—will affect your ability to fly. Reread FAR 91.17. It addresses not only alcohol consumption but also its after effects. Abusing alcohol can affect medical certification. Those who drink can have elevated blood pressure. Many doctors suspect alcoholism when blood pressure remains elevated despite other controlling measures. An ECG test conducted after a holiday party, for example, can indicate rhythm problems secondary to alcohol (caused by what is called the "holiday heart"). While not a significant problem, it may be a cause for a deferral of medical certification until proven otherwise. Alcohol can also affect blood tests, especially those indicating liver function. Although such tests are not a part of an FAA exam, many companies conduct these exams and may question the pilot.

Laws regarding DUI (driving under the influence) and DWI (driving while intoxicated) have become stricter in virtually all the states. Alcohol is metabolized out of the body rather quickly, but if you drink enough, there will still be alcohol on your breath and in your blood hours after your last drink. The police can stop you for any reasonable cause, such as a burned-out brake light, and if they even suspect that you have ingested alcohol recently, they will ticket you. That citation leads to thousands of dollars of expenses and fines, possible time in jail, impounding of your car, increased insurance rates, and a permanent record of your offense.

If you drink, be sure you have a designated driver to take you home and be sure you are alcohol-free before you show up for work or take a medical exam. New rules, effective January 1996, in the DOT'S "Alcohol Misuse Prevention Program" state that you cannot drink any alcohol (not just alcoholic beverages as stated in FAR 91.17) on the job or eight hours prior to beginning your job if it is a safety-sensitive operation, such as flying for a Part 121 or 135 operation. If you violate these rules, you will be reported to the Federal Air Surgeon, possibly lose your airman certification, and be fired if caught drinking alcohol on the job.

Remember, you must report any alcohol-related driving offense to the FAA within sixty days of the event and then report it at your next FAA medical examination.

OVER-THE-COUNTER MEDICATIONS

FAR 91.11(a)(3) states it is illegal to consume medicines that interfere with flying. Your physiological response to any medication, whether it is prescribed or over-the-counter, may be different at 5,000 feet than at sea level. Many medications sold over-the-counter are pain pills that include only aspirin, ibuprofen, Tylenol-like products, antihistamines, and stimulants. But those with ingredients that end in -*ine,* such as chlorpheniramine, phenylpropanolamine, or ephedrine and phenylephrine, may have a dangerous effect on you while you are flying. Trying to overcome the symptoms of a cold (which in itself should ground you temporarily) by taking antihistamines, which will make you drowsy, is an example of a seemingly small hazard that snowballs into a major one.

If there is any doubt, you should ground yourself. You are not qualified to play doctor and treat yourself, especially if you have an illness that can impair you in flight. Get into the habit of reading labels on over-the-counter medications to see what you are really taking. You will be surprised to find how many times a drug company combines caffeine, antihistamines, and decongestants, as well as alcohol and aspirin. A rule of thumb: if you have an illness or injury that you feel needs to be treated, then it is significant enough to ground yourself.

FATIGUE

To a pilot, fatigue is not just the result of overwork and long hours. Even though pilots are guaranteed so many hours of crew rest, trying to get a good night's sleep in a strange bed at odd hours is persistently difficult at best. And most pilots do not manage their rest periods effectively. There is no solution other than avoiding those factors that make it more difficult to sleep. The various techniques of relaxation therapy (e.g., transcendental meditation and biofeedback) have been very helpful for some pilots and may be worth reading about or discussing with a therapist. As I have mentioned, consumption of too much caffeine or alcohol prevents a truly restful sleep. Continuous noise is also fatiguing. The inactivity during a long, boring trip is fatiguing. Hours to which the body clock is unaccustomed lead to fatigue, and going from one time zone to another (jet lag) and coming back is also tiring—all from being unable to sleep and function at the usual time of day.

Some of these factors you can control, and some you can't. Your hours may be difficult to change, but you certainly don't have to have those four or five cups of coffee or the nightcap. Instead of going out with the crew before the turnaround the next day, get a good night's sleep. Drink plenty of water to avoid dehydration. And try to follow a schedule that is based on the fact that your body assumes you are back home. You will have to establish what you can tolerate: respect those factors that lead to increased fatigue, especially those you can control.

STRESS MANAGEMENT

Stress management is poorly understood by most people, especially flight crews. You may feel that you are immune to the stress of life, that you can cope with most every problem while controlling your emotions. However, your inability to cope with stress will begin to show up insidiously as poor weight control, increased blood pressure and pulse, unexplained headaches, fatigue, inability to do your job, and busted check rides. Your immune system suffers when you are under stress, preventing you from fighting off disease or recovering easily.

This is a major topic, but the only comment that I want to make is that if you are skeptical about counseling from psychologists and psychiatrists you must consider talking about your problems with somebody who can be objective, someone who is trained in analyzing your real problems—which may be different than those you perceive you have. The FAA does not consider this counseling medically disqualifying. If the treatment does not require medication and is not connected to alcohol or drug use, then this counseling does not have to be reported to the FAA.

FIRST AID ON TRIPS

Ear blocks. We discussed this in Chapter 4 in the section on hearing. Just remember to begin the Valsalva maneuver as soon as you notice any congestion. Don't wait until you are plugged up.

Constipation. This is almost invariably related to inactivity, dehydration, and the lack of bulk in your diet. Going through several time zones also throws off your schedule. This can usually be corrected by maintaining a good fluid intake and eating lots of "rabbit foods," such as celery, carrots, apples, and even prunes. In addition, you might try to establish more of a habit of following the "urge" rather than waiting until the end of the trip.

Diarrhea. This is often a result of the flu or indiscreet eating, and often there's very little you can do about it. If you are caught with this in the middle of a trip, stay away from all solid foods and drink mainly liquids until you return home. Trying further treatment by yourself may mask a more serious medical problem. Gastrointestinal problems are the leading cause of impairment on the flight deck.

Rectal itching. Sitting for long hours often creates a very uncomfortable irritation that may or may not be caused by hemorrhoids. More than likely it is a combination of sweating, hygiene, and poor quality toilet paper in the terminals. A product called "Tucks" is very beneficial; carry it in your flight bag. You should use it as supplement hygiene while on a trip and even put a fresh pad against your rectum if you are particularly uncomfortable. If the itching persists, you may have a very common yeast infection for which you can try some over-the-counter antifungal creams. If that fails, you should be examined by a doctor. In any case, persistent rectal itching is not something you should have to tolerate. It can be controlled.

Sore legs. Sore legs almost invariably are related to inactivity and poor venous circulation. Some tips to relieve sore legs are pushing and then relaxing both feet against the rudder pedals, wiggling your toes frequently, and getting up and moving around. Some people have poorer circulation than others and are therefore bothered more. Wearing good support hose (those that you buy in a drug store) is beneficial. Don't put up with the discomfort; this problem can degenerate to a more serious one, varicose veins. Try to correct the problem.

Colds and flu. Obviously you shouldn't fly if you have a serious cold or the flu, but sometimes you become sick in the middle of a trip. If there is any way that you can, ground yourself and deadhead back. If you can't, stay away from medications because they will only make things worse. For congestion, keep a small bottle of nasal spray (the long-lasting, quick-acting kind) in your flight bag. This can be used as a "get-you-down" treatment and should be used only for that purpose. Don't get in the habit of using it to allow you to fly with a cold or congestion. Also, follow a liquid diet and pass responsibilities to your colleagues. You can't cure a cold or the flu, and you can't eliminate symptoms without creating more, despite what the ads say.

RETIREMENT

Much has been written about the age sixty rule. Historically, it is more of a problem for a vocal minority than the silent majority of pilots who choose to retire at that age. In any case, the age sixty rule is not a medical standard; it's a rule found in Part 121. An AME and the FAA cannot waive that rule no matter what they find on a medical exam. Age sixty is arbitrary, but what is a better age? We all recognize that with age come changes, physiological (e.g., vision, reaction time, tolerance to illness) and psychological (e.g., cognitive thinking and short-term memory loss). What tests would prove that older pilots are still competent? And extending the age limit means additional testing, even for pilots who are under age sixty.

So the age sixty rule is a complex medical, administrative, and financial issue not easily resolved. In fact, it's two issues: how age can be used as a medical parameter without being discriminatory and how to gauge the effects of aging. We all know as we get older we experience changes, unpredictable and often untestable. Although there is increased interest in changing this rule, a final disposition by the FAA came out in early 1996 that essentially stated there was not enough evidence to change the rule and until cost-effective and reliable testing could be developed to determine any impairment from aging the FAA would not accept any more appeals.

Finally, I would like to make a few comments about retirement, whether you have to retire medically or you are forced to at age sixty. This is something that very few pilots think about, especially in terms of preparation. If you are fortunate enough to maintain your health until you are age sixty, what are you going to do with this good health? What happens if you have to retire because of some medical problem that is beyond your control? Take the time to dream about what you would like to do, especially since you already know you are going to have to retire at this age. Consider turning a hobby into an income-producing business, a vocation you could always fall back on, and start planning it now, even if you're in your thirties.

If you should happen to see a course in an adult education program that interests you, go ahead and take it instead of just thinking about it. Talk with your retired friends about what they're doing. Those fringe benefits of retirement and disability pay are not going to be the answer. The philosophy "I've paid my dues and now I can play" just doesn't work because without meaningful activity you fall apart. Besides, some pilots find flying less than challenging as they get older. One of the things I have found in the aviation community is that often when pilots medically retire or retire at age sixty they feel lost. Remember, you will be in that situation someday, so keep in touch with the retired and find out what they are doing. I have seen too many pilots grounded unexpectedly who literally waste away because they have nothing to do. They have not planned ahead and are unable to cope with being grounded.

IN REVIEW

When anyone is confronted with a serious illness, that person will understandably use different methods of denial initially, such as putting off seeking help, second-guessing the diagnosis and therapy of the doctor, and looking for any way out, even to the extent of going to quacks for therapy. Professional pilots who have careers at stake, and even recreational pilots, are more subject to denial, even to the point of sacrificing their health to maintain their certification. This is understandable but unrealistic.

If, in fact, you have a disorder that will keep you from flying, the sooner you find out about it, the sooner you can look for an alternative career and then more easily accept the fate of your illness. Unfortunately most professional pilots consider flying to be the only desirable work. As a result, a pilot who has not even considered a second career cannot and often will not accept a disqualifying illness—or a mandatory age sixty retirement. Accept the fact that you are less likely to fulfill your professional dream than most people—because nonpilots can return to work after a heart attack or the day after they turn sixty. Being prepared for the odds of losing your medical certificate will make you less defensive about that unexpected disqualifying illness and allow your doctor the opportunity to help you with all your careers, including flying.

Nothing that I have written in this chapter has been new to you, but I do want you to put these matters in proper perspective. Hopefully, being a healthy, safe pilot with a current medical certificate is more important than those abuses I have described. Any one of these problems alone is probably insignificant. If you start combining them, then you are going to run into trouble. Very few pilots are grounded for reasons that were caused solely by events beyond their control. You have four standards of health. The first is that state of health that you desire. The second is that state of health that your doctor desires. The third is that state of health that the FAA requires to certify you. The fourth is that state of health that you must have while you are flying. All four could be different and have different consequences for you and your career.

Keep these things in mind. You may be allowed to fly under relaxed medical restrictions, but you will ultimately be responsible if you have a medical problem in flight. Consider your responsibility to your passengers and then the liability of an accident if you intend to fly when you know you should not.

Appendix I

Part 67 of Federal Air Regulations: Medical Standards and Certification

The following is a definition of the regulations that your AME and the FAA will use to pass judgment on you and your medical certificate (these rules became effective September 16, 1996). They are relatively easy to read and essentially self-explanatory. My interpretations and explanations, when appropriate, are in brackets. A more definitive interpretation of these standards can be found in the Guide for Aviation Medical Examiners, which is used by these doctors to assist in determining if a pilot meets the intent of Part 67. An overview of this guide with a brief explanation for use by pilots is found in Appendix II.

Everything is potentially certifiable *if* it can be proven that you are not a risk in flight. The new regulations are meant to be more specific in some situations and less restrictive in others. They still require judgment calls by AMEs and FAA flight surgeons. In addition, Part 61 has been revised to incorporate the third-class three-year duration. Otherwise, there is little difference between the three classes of medical certification except for the ECG and the more comprehensive near vision test required for first-class medical certification.

Subpart B—First-Class Airman Medical Certificate
[Note: Except for the ECG, the following are about the same for Second Class].

§ 67.101 Eligibility.

To be eligible for a first-class airman medical certificate, and to remain eligible for a first-class airman medical certificate, a person must meet the requirements of this subpart.

§ 67.103 Eye.

Eye standards for a first-class airman medical certificate are:
(a) Distant visual acuity of 20/20 or better in each eye separately, with or without corrective lenses. If corrective lenses (spectacles or contact lenses) are necessary for 20/20 vision, the person may be eligible only on the condition that corrective lenses are worn while exercising the privileges of an airman certificate. [Note: There is no longer an uncorrected distant vision

standard. In other words, a waiver is no longer necessary for vision in excess of 20/100 as long as it is corrected to 20/20 using conventional means.]

(b) Near vision of 20/40 or better, Snellen equivalent, at 16 inches in each eye separately, with or without corrective lenses. If age 50 or older, near vision of 20/40 or better, Snellen equivalent, at both 16 inches and 32 inches in each eye separately, with or without corrective lenses. [Note: The age 50 requirement takes into account that your near vision will deteriorate, especially for focal lengths where you must read something at sixteen inches and then visualize the panel at thirty-two inches. Without the ability to correct, your vision will be severely impaired, especially at night when you are already fatigued and hypoxic. The guidelines state that your vision is acceptable if it can be corrected to 20/40 or better. This is not a requirement for third class.]

(c) Ability to perceive those colors necessary for the safe performance of airman duties. [Note: This leaves much to the discretion of the AME and the FAA, regardless of what your score is. Once again, the guidelines will establish what is expected, and they are essentially unchanged. Conventional testing will be used, as before, as well as the Statement of Demonstrated Ability (SODA) or a medical check ride.]

(d) Normal fields of vision.

(e) No acute or chronic pathological condition of either eye or adnexae that interferes with the proper function of an eye, that may reasonably be expected to progress to that degree, or that may reasonably be expected to be aggravated by flying.

(f) Bifoveal fixation and vergence-phoria relationship sufficient to prevent a break in fusion under conditions that may reasonably be expected to occur in performing airman duties. Tests for the factors named in this paragraph are not required except for persons found to have more than 1 prism diopter of hyperphoria, 6 prism diopters of esophoria, or 6 prism diopters of exophoria. If any of these values are exceeded, the Federal Air Surgeon may require the person to be examined by a qualified eye specialist to determine if there is bifoveal fixation and an adequate vergence-phoria relationship. However, if otherwise eligible, the person is issued a medical certificate pending the results of the examination. [Note: The problem here is your ability to fuse both eyes when focusing on a distant object. If there is a weakness and your eyes are unable to maintain fusion, you experience double vision, especially when you are fatigued or hypoxic.]

§ 67.105 Ear, nose, throat, and equilibrium.

Ear, nose, throat, and equilibrium standards for a first-class airman medical certificate are:

(a) The person shall demonstrate acceptable hearing by at least one of the following tests:

(1) Demonstrate an ability to hear an average conversational voice in a quiet room, using both ears, at a distance of 6 feet from the examiner, with the back turned to the examiner.

(2) Demonstrate an acceptable understanding of speech as determined by audiometric speech discrimination testing to a score of at least 70 percent obtained in one ear or in a sound field environment.

(3) Provide acceptable results of pure tone audiometric testing of unaided hearing acuity according to the following table of worst acceptable thresholds, using the calibration standards of the American National Standards Institute, 1969:

FREQUENCY (Hz)	500 Hz	1000 Hz	2000 Hz	3000 Hz
Better ear (Db)	35	30	30	40
Poorer ear (Db)	35	50	50	60

(b) No disease or condition of the middle or internal ear, nose, oral cavity, pharynx, or larynx that—

(1) Interferes with, or is aggravated by, flying or may reasonably be expected to do so; or

(2) Interferes with, or may reasonably be expected to interfere with, clear and effective speech communication.

(c) No disease or condition manifested by, or that may reasonably be expected to be manifested by, vertigo or a disturbance of equilibrium.

§ 67.107 Mental.

Mental standards for a first-class airman medical certificate are:

(a) No established medical history or clinical diagnosis of any of the following:

(1) A personality disorder that is severe enough to have repeatedly manifested itself by overt acts.

(2) A psychosis. As used in this section, "psychosis" refers to a mental disorder in which:

(i) The individual has manifested delusions, hallucinations, grossly bizarre or disorganized behavior, or other commonly accepted symptoms of this condition; or

(ii) The individual may reasonably be expected to manifest delusions, hallucinations, grossly bizarre or disorganized behavior, or other commonly accepted symptoms of this condition.

(3) A bipolar disorder. [Note: Same as manic-depression.]

(4) Substance dependence, except where there is established clinical evidence, satisfactory to the Federal Air Surgeon, of recovery, including sustained total abstinence from the substance(s) for not less than the preceding 2 years. As used in this section—

(i) "Substance" includes: alcohol; other sedatives and hypnotics; anxiolytics; opioids; central nervous system stimulants such as cocaine, amphetamines, and similarly acting sympathomimetics; hallucinogens; phencyclidine or similarly acting arylcyclohexylamines; cannabis; inhalants; and other psychoactive drugs and chemicals; and

(ii) "Substance dependence" means a condition in which a person is dependent on a substance, other than tobacco or ordinary xanthine-containing (e.g., caffeine) beverages, as evidenced by—

(A) Increased tolerance;

(B) Manifestation of withdrawal symptoms;

(C) Impaired control of use; or

(D) Continued use despite damage to physical health or impairment of social, personal, or occupational functioning.

(b) No substance abuse within the preceding 2 years defined as:

(1) Use of a substance in a situation in which that use was physically hazardous, if there has been at any other time an instance of the use of a substance also in a situation in which that use was physically hazardous;

(2) A verified positive drug test result acquired under an anti-drug program or internal program of the U.S. Department of Transportation or any other Administration within the U.S. Department of Transportation; or [Note: This is new but in tune with other laws and policies in the aviation industry.]

(3) Misuse of a substance that the Federal Air Surgeon, based on case history and appropriate, qualified medical judgment relating to the substance involved, finds—

(i) Makes the person unable to safely perform the duties or exercise the privileges of the airman certificate applied for or held; or

(ii) May reasonably be expected, for the maximum duration of the airman medical certificate applied for or held, to make the person unable to perform those duties or exercise those privileges.

(c) No other personality disorder, neurosis, or other mental condition that the Federal Air Surgeon, based on the case history and appropriate, qualified medical judgment relating to the condition involved, finds—

(1) Makes the person unable to safely perform the duties or exercise the privileges of the airman certificate applied for or held; or

(2) May reasonably be expected, for the maximum duration of the airman medical certificate applied for or held, to make the person unable to perform those duties or exercise those privileges. [Note: This can be a very subjective regulation, difficult to clearly define, diagnose, and document.

However, it does allow the Federal Air Surgeon to review each case on an individual basis so that a pilot with these conditions can be considered under the special issuance policy stated below.]

§ 67.109 Neurologic.

Neurologic standards for a first-class airman medical certificate are:

(a) No established medical history or clinical diagnosis of any of the following:

(1) Epilepsy;

(2) A disturbance of consciousness without satisfactory medical explanation of the cause; or

(3) A transient loss of control of nervous system function(s) without satisfactory medical explanation of the cause.

(b) No other seizure disorder, disturbance of consciousness, or neurologic condition that the Federal Air Surgeon, based on the case history and appropriate, qualified medical judgment relating to the condition involved, finds—

(1) Makes the person unable to safely perform the duties or exercise the privileges of the airman certificate applied for or held; or

(2) May reasonably be expected, for the maximum duration of the airman medical certificate applied for or held, to make the person unable to perform those duties or exercise those privileges.

§ 67.111 Cardiovascular.

Cardiovascular standards for a first-class airman medical certificate are:

(a) No established medical history or clinical diagnosis of any of the following:

(1) Myocardial infarction;

(2) Angina pectoris;

(3) Coronary heart disease that has required treatment or, if untreated, that has been symptomatic or clinically significant;

(4) Cardiac valve replacement;

(5) Permanent cardiac pacemaker implantation; or

(6) Heart replacement.

(b) A person applying for first-class medical certification must demonstrate an absence of myocardial infarction and other clinically significant abnormality on electrocardiographic examination:

(1) At the first application after reaching the 35th birthday; and

(2) On an annual basis after reaching the 40th birthday.

(c) An electrocardiogram will satisfy a requirement of paragraph (b) of this section if it is dated no earlier than 60 days before the date of the application it is to accompany and was performed and transmitted according to acceptable standards and techniques.

§ 67.113 General medical condition.

The general medical standards for a first-class airman medical certificate are:

(a) No established medical history or clinical diagnosis of diabetes mellitus that requires insulin or any other hypoglycemic drug for control.

(b) No other organic, functional, or structural disease, defect, or limitation that the Federal Air Surgeon, based on the case history and appropriate, qualified medical judgment relating to the condition involved, finds—

(1) Makes the person unable to safely perform the duties or exercise the privileges of the airman certificate applied for or held; or

(2) May reasonably be expected, for the maximum duration of the airman medical certificate applied for or held, to make the person unable to perform those duties or exercise those privileges.

(c) No medication or other treatment that the Federal Air Surgeon, based on the case history and appropriate, qualified medical judgment relating to the medication or other treatment involved, finds—

(1) Makes the person unable to safely perform the duties or exercise the privileges of the airman certificate applied for or held; or

(2) May reasonably be expected, for the maximum duration of the airman medical certificate applied for or held, to make the person unable to perform those duties or exercise those privileges.

§ 67.115 Discretionary issuance.

A person who does not meet the provisions of §§ 67.103 through 67.113 may apply for the discretionary issuance of a certificate under § 67.401.

Subpart E—Certification Procedures

§ 67.401 Special issuance of medical certificates.

[Note: The following are self-explanatory, one of the improvements over the previous edition of the regulations. Any item that could be misunderstood is explained in these "Notes."]

(a) At the discretion of the Federal Air Surgeon, an Authorization for Special Issuance of a Medical Certificate (Authorization), valid for a specified period, may be granted to a person who does not meet the provisions of subparts B, C, or D of this part if the person shows to the satisfaction of the Federal Air Surgeon that the duties authorized by the class of medical certificate applied for can be performed without endangering public safety during the period in which the Authorization would be in force. The Federal Air Surgeon may authorize a special medical flight test, practical test, or medical evaluation for this purpose. A medical certificate of the appropriate class may be issued to a person who does not meet the provisions of subparts of this part if that person possesses a valid Authorization and is otherwise eligible. An airman medical certificate issued in accordance with this section shall expire no later than the end of the validity period or upon the withdrawal of the Authorization upon which it is based. At the end of its specified validity period, for grant of a new Authorization, the person must again show to the satisfaction of the Federal Air Surgeon that the duties authorized by the class of medical certificate applied for can be performed without endangering public safety during the period in which the Authorization would be in force.

(b) At the discretion of the Federal Air Surgeon, a Statement of Demonstrated Ability (SODA) may be granted, instead of an Authorization, to a person whose disqualifying condition is static or nonprogressive and who has been found capable of performing airman duties without endangering public safety. A SODA does not expire and authorizes a designated aviation medical examiner to issue a medical certificate of a specified class if the examiner finds that the condition described on its face has not adversely changed.

(c) In granting an Authorization or SODA, the Federal Air Surgeon may consider the person's operational experience and any medical facts that may affect the ability of the person to perform airman duties including—

(1) The combined effect on the person of failure to meet more than one requirement of this part; and

(2) The prognosis derived from professional consideration of all available information regarding the person.

(d) In granting an Authorization or SODA under this section, the Federal Air Surgeon specifies the class of medical certificate authorized to be issued and may do any or all of the following:

(1) Limit the duration of an Authorization;

(2) Condition the granting of a new Authorization on the results of subsequent medical tests, examinations, or evaluations;

(3) State on the Authorization or SODA, and any medical certificate based upon it, any operational limitation needed for safety; or

(4) Condition the continued effect of an Authorization or SODA, and any second- or third-class medical certificate based upon it, on compliance with a statement of functional limitations issued to the person in coordina-

tion with the Director of Flight Standards or the Director's designee. [Note: This is where the FAA can add an operational limitation to allow medical certification, but not in the case of first-class certification.]

(e) In determining whether an Authorization or SODA should be granted to an applicant for a third-class medical certificate, the Federal Air Surgeon considers the freedom of an airman, exercising the privileges of a private pilot certificate, to accept reasonable risks to his or her person and property that are not acceptable in the exercise of commercial or airline transport pilot privileges, and, at the same time, considers the need to protect the safety of persons and property in other aircraft and on the ground. [Note: This allows the FAA more flexibility for certifying noncommercial pilots with significant medical problems. The FAA anticipates that pilots will use good judgment in determining if they meet the requirements of FAR 61.53, which states a pilot is not legal if he or she has a known medical deficiency. See Chapter 2.]

(f) An Authorization or SODA granted under the provisions of this section to a person who does not meet the applicable provisions of subparts B, C, or D of this part may be withdrawn, at the discretion of the Federal Air Surgeon, at any time if—

(1) There is adverse change in the holder's medical condition;

(2) The holder fails to comply with a statement of functional limitations or operational limitations issued as a condition of certification under this section;

(3) Public safety would be endangered by the holder's exercise of airman privileges;

(4) The holder fails to provide medical information reasonably needed by the Federal Air Surgeon for certification under this section; or

(5) The holder makes or causes to be made a statement or entry that is the basis for withdrawal of an Authorization or SODA under § 67.403.

(g) A person who has been granted an Authorization or SODA under this section based on a special medical flight or practical test need not take the test again during later physical examinations unless the Federal Air Surgeon determines or has reason to believe that the physical deficiency has or may have degraded to a degree to require another special medical flight test or practical test.

(h) The authority of the Federal Air Surgeon under this section is also exercised by the Manager, Aeromedical Certification Division, and each Regional Flight Surgeon.

(i) If an Authorization or SODA is withdrawn under paragraph (f) of this section the following procedures apply:

(1) The holder of the Authorization or SODA will be served a letter of withdrawal, stating the reason for the action;

(2) By not later than 60 days after the service of the letter of with-

drawal, the holder of the Authorization or SODA may request, in writing, that the Federal Air Surgeon provide for review of the decision to withdraw. The request for review may be accompanied by supporting medical evidence;

(3) Within 60 days of receipt of a request for review, a written final decision either affirming or reversing the decision to withdraw will be issued; and

(4) A medical certificate rendered invalid pursuant to a withdrawal, in accordance with paragraph (a) of this section, shall be surrendered to the Administrator upon request.

(j) No grant of a special issuance made prior to September 16, 1996, may be used to obtain a medical certificate after the earlier of the following dates:

(1) September 16, 1997; or

(2) The date on which the holder of such special issuance is required to provide additional information to the FAA as a condition for continued medical certification.

§ 67.409 Denial of medical certificate.

(a) Any person who is denied a medical certificate by an aviation medical examiner may, within 30 days after the date of the denial, apply in writing and in duplicate to the Federal Air Surgeon, Attention: Manager, Aeromedical Certification Division, AAM-300, Federal Aviation Administration, P.O. Box 26080, Oklahoma City, Oklahoma 73126, for reconsideration of that denial. If the person does not ask for reconsideration during the 30-day period after the date of the denial, he or she is considered to have withdrawn the application for a medical certificate. [Note: This doesn't mean the door is permanently closed if you don't respond in thirty days. It means the application is withdrawn and filed, instead of being held in a pending file. When you send additional information to request reconsideration, the file is reopened.]

(b) The denial of a medical certificate—

(1) By an aviation medical examiner is not a denial by the Administrator under 49 U.S.C. 44703. [Note: In other words, the denial by the AME is not final and is subject to review with either confirmation of denial or recertification.]

(2) By the Federal Air Surgeon is considered to be a denial by the Administrator under 49 U.S.C. 44703.

(3) By the Manager, Aeromedical Certification Division, or a Regional Flight Surgeon is considered to be a denial by the Administrator under 49 U.S.C. 44703 except where the person does not meet the standards of §§ 67.107(b)(3) and (c), 67.109(b), or 67.113(b) and (c); 67.207(b)(3) and (c), 67.209(b), or 67.213(b) and (c); or 67.307(b)(3) and (c), 67.309(b), or

67.313(b) and (c). [Note: These include the mandatory standards for denial and are subject to being considered under 67.401, special issuance of medical certificates.]

(c) Any action taken under § 67.407(c) that wholly or partly reverses the issue of a medical certificate by an aviation medical examiner is the denial of a medical certificate under paragraph (b) of this section.

(d) If the issue of a medical certificate is wholly or partly reversed by the Federal Air Surgeon; the Manager, Aeromedical Certification Division; or a Regional Flight Surgeon, the person holding that certificate shall surrender it, upon request of the FAA.

§ 67.413 Medical records.

(a) Whenever the Administrator finds that additional medical information or history is necessary to determine whether an applicant for or the holder of a medical certificate meets the medical standards for it, the Administrator requests that person to furnish that information or to authorize any clinic, hospital, physician, or other person to release to the Administrator all available information or records concerning that history. If the applicant or holder fails to provide the requested medical information or history or to authorize the release so requested, the Administrator may suspend, modify, or revoke all medical certificates the airman holds or may, in the case of an applicant, deny the application for an airman medical certificate.

(b) If an airman medical certificate is suspended or modified under paragraph (a) of this section, that suspension or modification remains in effect until the requested information, history, or authorization is provided to the FAA and until the Federal Air Surgeon determines whether the person meets the medical standards under this part.

These regulations were signed by David R. Hinson, FAA administrator. They were issued in Washington, D.C., on March 12, 1996.

The FAA must apply FAR Part 67 to everyone, regardless of proficiency, type of flying, or number of hours. In other words, you are considered unsafe if you have an unacceptable medical problem unless you can prove otherwise. FAR Part 67 allows the FAA's Federal Air Surgeon to consider additional information that indicates you are still safe even if you don't meet the "letter of the law." It's essential that you at least respect the intent of these standards and understand that everything is potentially certifiable, if you follow the procedures outlined here.

Appendix ▌▌

Overview of the FAA's *Guide for Aviation Medical Examiners*

The information in this appendix is extracted from the September 1996 *Guide for Aviation Medical Examiners.* Only the more common conditions and disorders that affect medical certification are covered in this abridged version. Keep in mind that the guide is intended for the AME. Still, it will give you an idea of what to expect from the FAA and your AME. For clarification of any of these issues, or to read the full guide, you should consult your AME.

APPLICATION FOR MEDICAL CERTIFICATION

The following section covers what the AME looks for in the pilot's portion of the Application Form 8500-8.

General Information

The applicant must personally enter all data and make all corrections on the application form. The applicant should initial all corrections. The application constitutes a legal document and must be completed in the applicant's handwriting. Strict compliance with this procedure is essential in case it becomes necessary for the FAA to take legal action for falsification of the application.

The following relates to the history items on the front of Form 8500-8.

ITEM 17. DO YOU CURRENTLY USE ANY MEDICATION (PRESCRIPTION OR NONPRESCRIPTION)?

If the applicant checks yes, the name, dosage, frequency, and purpose of each medication should be reported. This includes both prescription and non-prescription medication. During periods in which the foregoing medications are being used for treatment of acute illnesses, the airman is under obligation not to perform the duties of an airman unless cleared by the FAA.

ITEM 18. MEDICAL HISTORY [The pilot must respond affirmatively if at any time the following disorders occur.]

18.a. *Frequent or severe headaches.* A history of headaches without seque-lae is not disqualifying. Some require only temporary disqualification during periods when the headaches are likely to occur or require treatment. Other types of headaches may preclude certification by the Examiner and require special evaluation and consideration (e.g., migraine and cluster headaches).

18.b. *Dizziness or fainting spells.* One or two episodes of dizziness or even fainting may not be disqualifying. For example, dizziness upon suddenly aris-ing when ill is not a true dysfunction. Likewise, the orthostatic faint associ-ated with moderate anemia is no threat to aviation safety as long as the individual is temporarily disqualified until the anemia is corrected. Episodic disorders of dizziness or disequilibrium, however, are another matter and re-quire careful evaluation and consideration by the FAA.

18.c. *Unconsciousness for any reason.* An unexplained disturbance of con-sciousness is disqualifying under the medical standards. Because a distur-bance of consciousness may be expected to be totally incapacitating, individuals with such histories pose a high risk to safety and must be denied or deferred by the Examiner. If the cause of the disturbance is explained and a loss of consciousness is not likely to recur, then medical certification may be possible.

18.d. *Eye or vision trouble except glasses.* The Examiner should personally explore the applicant's history by asking questions concerning any changes in vision, unusual visual experiences (halos, scintillations, etc.), sensitivity to light, injuries, surgery, or current use of medication. Is there a history of se-rious eye disease such as glaucoma or other disease commonly associated with secondary eye changes, such as diabetes?

18.e. *Hay fever or allergy.* Hay fever controlled solely by desensitization with-out requiring antihistamines or other medications is not disqualifying. Indi-viduals who have hay fever that requires only occasional seasonal therapy may be certified by the Examiner with the stipulation that they not fly during the time when symptoms occur and treatment is required. However, nonse-dating antihistamines including loratadine, astemizole, or terfenadine may be used while flying, after adequate individual experience has determined that the medication is well tolerated without significant side effects. In the case of severe allergies, the Examiner should deny or defer certification and provide a report to the Aeromedical Certification Division, AAM-300, that details the period and duration of symptoms and the nature and dosage of drugs used for treatment and/or prevention.

18.f. *Asthma or lung disease.* A history of mild or seasonal asthmatic symptoms is not disqualifying if the applicant otherwise meets the medical standards and currently requires no treatment. A history of frequent severe attacks is disqualifying. Certificate issuance may be possible in other cases. If additional information is obtained, it must be submitted to the FAA. A history of a single episode of spontaneous pneumothorax is considered disqualifying for airman medical certification until there is x-ray evidence of resolution and until it can be determined that no condition that would be likely to cause recurrence is present. On the other hand, an individual who has sustained a repeat pneumothorax normally is not eligible for certification until surgical intervention is carried out to correct the underlying problem. A person who has such a history is usually able to resume airman duties 3 months after the surgery. If the applicant has frequent exacerbations or any degree of exertional dyspnea (trouble breathing), certification should be deferred.

18.g. *Heart or vascular trouble.* Because of the possibility of sudden and severe incapacitation, certain heart conditions are disqualifying based upon history alone, regardless of how remote that history may be. Part 67 provides that, for all classes of medical certificates, an established medical history or clinical diagnosis of myocardial infarction, angina pectoris, cardiac valve replacement, permanent cardiac pacemaker implantation, heart replacement, or coronary heart disease that has required treatment or, if untreated, that has been symptomatic or clinically significant is cause for denial. The Examiner may not issue a certificate to a person with such a history unless specifically authorized to do so by the FAA. The Examiner may issue a letter of denial or defer issuance and forward the application to the Manager of the Aeromedical Certification Division, AAM-300. The Examiner should report any available information concerning this history in Item 60 of the application form.

The Examiner should deny or defer issuance to any applicant with a history of arrhythmia, except when the disturbance is sinus arrhythmia or occasional ventricular ectopic beats not due to organic heart disease. An airman who has had an episode of acute rhythm disturbance may be considered by the Federal Air Surgeon for medical certification under the special issuance section of Part 67 after an acceptable interval without recurrence. A history of cardioversion or drug treatment, per se, does not rule out certification. A current, complete cardiovascular evaluation will be required. An individual with chronic rhythm disturbance may apply for medical certification and would require a similar evaluation.

18.h. *High or low blood pressure.* Issuance of a medical certificate to an applicant with high blood pressure may depend on the current blood pressure levels and whether the applicant is taking antihypertensive medication. The Examiner should also determine if the applicant has a history of complications, adverse reactions to therapy, hospitalization, etc.

18.i. *Stomach, liver, or intestinal trouble.* A history of acute gastrointestinal disorders is usually not disqualifying once recovery is achieved. Many chronic gastrointestinal diseases may preclude issuance of a medical certificate (e.g., cirrhosis, chronic hepatitis, malignancy, ulcerative colitis). Colostomy following surgery for cancer may be allowed by the FAA with special follow-up reports. The Examiner should not issue a medical certificate if the applicant has a recent history of bleeding ulcers. Otherwise, ulcers must not have been active within the past 3 months.

18.j. *Kidney stone or blood in urine.* An Examiner may not issue a medical certificate to an applicant with a history of recent or recurring renal stones unless there is documentation that there is no residual stone or significant likelihood of recurrence. If the applicant has a remote history of a single episode of a kidney stone and is free of signs or symptoms, the Examiner may issue a medical certificate. A history of recent or significant hematuria (blood in the urine) requires further elaboration or evaluation.

18.k. *Diabetes.* A medical history or clinical diagnosis of diabetes mellitus requiring insulin or other hypoglycemic drugs for control are disqualifying. The application of persons with a history of diabetes currently treated by hypoglycemic medication should be deferred and forwarded to the Aeromedical Certification Division, AAM-300, for further evaluation. The Examiner can help expedite the FAA review by assisting the applicant in gathering medical records and submitting a current specialty report. The application of persons with a history of diabetes controlled by diet and exercise may be issued a medical certificate by the Examiner in accordance with the guidelines. [This has been revised as of December 1996. See Appendix III. Check with your AME about the current status of the standards for pilots using insulin.]

18.l. *Neurological disorders: epilepsy, seizures, stroke, paralysis, etc.* An established diagnosis of epilepsy, a transient loss of control of nervous system function(s) without satisfactory medical explanation of the cause, or a disturbance of consciousness without a satisfactory medical explanation of the cause is a basis for denial no matter how remote the history. A medical certificate should be denied or deferred if the applicant has a history of or an existing neurological condition or disease that may be incapacitating. This includes a history of seizures or a single seizure. Although the likelihood for certification is poor, the Examiner can assist the applicant who wishes further consideration by helping to acquire all past records.

18.m. *Mental disorders of any sort: depression, anxiety, etc.* An affirmative answer to Item 18.m. requires investigation through supplemental history taking. Dispositions will vary according to the details obtained. An applicant with an established history of a personality disorder that is severe enough to have repeatedly manifested itself by overt acts, a psychosis disorder, or a bipolar disorder must be denied or deferred by the Examiner.

18.n. *Substance dependence; or failed a drug test ever; or substance abuse or use of illegal substance in the last 5 years.* In the future item 18.n. of FAA Form 8500-8 will be revised to read "in the last 2 years." Until revised, however, the current wording requiring a 5-year history should be followed. "Substance" includes alcohol and other drugs (i.e., PCP, sedatives, and hypnotics; anxiolytics; marijuana; cocaine; opioids; amphetamines; hallucinogens; and other psychoactive drugs or chemicals). For a "yes" answer to Item 18.n., the Examiner should obtain a detailed description of the history. A history of substance dependence or substance abuse is disqualifying. The Examiner must defer issuance of a certificate if there is doubt concerning an applicant's substance use.

18.o. *Alcohol dependence or abuse.* See Item 18.n.

18.p. *Suicide attempt.* A history of suicidal attempts or suicidal gestures requires further evaluation. The ultimate decision of whether an applicant with such a history is eligible for medical certification rests with the FAA.

18.q. *Motion sickness requiring medication.* A careful supplemental history is indicated when the applicant responds affirmatively to this item. Because motion sickness varies with the nature of the stimulus, it is most helpful to know if the problem has occurred in flight or under similar circumstances. If in doubt or if medication is repeatedly required, the Examiner should deny or defer issuance.

18.r. *Military medical discharge.* If the person has received a military medical discharge, the Examiner should take additional history and record it. It is helpful to know the circumstances surrounding the discharge, including dates, and whether the individual is receiving disability compensation. If the applicant is receiving veteran's disability benefits, the claim number and service number are helpful in obtaining copies of pertinent medical records. The fact that the applicant is receiving disability benefits does not necessarily mean that the application should be denied.

18.s. *Medical rejection by military service.* The Examiner should inquire about the place, cause, and date of rejection and enter the information. It is of great assistance to the applicant and the FAA if the Examiner can help obtain copies of military documents for attachment to the FAA Form 8500-8. Disposition will depend upon whether the medical condition still exists or whether a history of such a condition requires denial or deferral under the FAA medical standards.

18.t. *Rejection for life or health insurance.* The Examiner should inquire regarding the circumstances of rejection. Disposition will depend upon whether the medical condition still exists or whether a history of such a condition requires denial or deferral under the FAA medical standards.

18.u. *Admission to hospital.* For each admission, the applicant should list the dates, diagnoses, duration, treatment, name of the attending physician, and complete address of the hospital or clinic. If previously reported, the applicant may enter "previously reported, no change." A history of hospitalization does not disqualify an applicant, although the medical condition that resulted in hospitalization may.

18.v. *Conviction and/or Administrative Action History.* The events to be reported are specifically identified in Item 18.v. of FAA Form 8500-8. If "yes" is checked, the applicant must describe the conviction(s) and/or administrative action(s) in the EXPLANATIONS box. The description must include:

- The alcohol or drug offense for which the applicant was convicted or the type of administrative action involved (e.g., attendance at an alcohol treatment program in lieu of conviction; license denial, suspension, cancellation, or revocation for refusal to be tested; educational safe driving program for multiple speeding convictions; etc.);
- The name of the state or other jurisdiction involved; and
- The date of the conviction and/or administrative action.

If there have been no new convictions or administrative actions since the last application, the applicant may enter "previously reported, no change." Convictions and/or administrative actions affecting driving privileges may raise questions about the applicant's fitness for certification and may be cause for disqualification. A single driving while intoxicated (DWI) conviction or administrative action usually is not cause for denial if there are no other instances or indications of substance dependence or abuse. The Examiner should inquire regarding the applicant's alcohol use history, the circumstances surrounding the incident, and document those findings.

NOTE: It should be noted that the airman's reporting of alcohol or drug offenses (i.e., motor vehicle action) on the history part of the medical application does not relieve the airman of responsibility to report each motor vehicle action to the FAA; Civil Aviation Security Division, AAC-700; P.O. Box 25810; Oklahoma City, OK 73125-0810.

18.w. *History of nontraffic convictions.* The applicant must report any other (nontraffic) convictions (e.g., assault, battery, public intoxication, robbery, etc.). The applicant must name the charge for which convicted and the date of the conviction(s) in the EXPLANATIONS box.

18.x. *Other illness, disability, or surgery.* The applicant should describe the nature of these illnesses in the EXPLANATIONS box. If additional records, tests, or specialty reports are necessary in order to make a certification decision, the applicant should be so advised. If the applicant does not wish to provide the information requested by the Examiner, the Examiner should defer issuance.

If the applicant wishes to have the FAA review the application and decide what ancillary documentation is needed, the Examiner should defer issuance of the medical certificate and forward the completed FAA Form 8500-8 to the FAA. If the Examiner proceeds to obtain documentation, but all data will not be received within 2 weeks, FAA Form 8500-8 should be sent immediately to the Aeromedical Certification Division, AAM-300, with a note that additional documents will be forwarded later under separate cover.

ITEM 19. VISITS TO HEALTH PROFESSIONAL WITHIN LAST 3 YEARS

The applicant should list all visits in the last 3 years to a physician, physician assistant, nurse, nurse practitioner, psychologist, clinical social worker, or substance abuse specialist for treatment, examination, or medical/mental evaluation. The applicant should list visits for counseling only if related to a personal substance dependence or abuse or psychiatric condition. The applicant should give the name, date, address, and type of health professional consulted and briefly state the reason for the consultation. Multiple visits to one health professional for the same condition may be aggregated on one line. Routine dental, eye, and FAA periodic medical examinations and consultations with an employer-sponsored employee assistance program (EAP) may be excluded unless the consultations were for the applicant's substance dependence or abuse or unless the consultations resulted in referral for psychiatric evaluation or treatment.

If an explanation has been given on previous report(s) and there has been no change in the condition, the applicant may enter "previously reported, no change."

Of particular importance is the reporting of conditions that have developed since the applicant's last FAA medical examination. The Examiner is asked to comment on all entries, including those "previously reported, no change." These comments may be entered under Item 60 or placed on a supplemental sheet and attached to FAA Form 8500-8.

ITEM 20. APPLICANT'S NATIONAL DRIVER REGISTER AND CERTIFYING DECLARATIONS

In addition to making a declaration of the completeness and truthfulness of the applicant's responses on the medical application, the Applicant's Declaration authorizes the National Driver Register to release the applicant's adverse driving history information, if any, to the FAA. The FAA uses such information to verify information provided in the application. The applicant should be instructed to sign Item 20 after reading the declaration. The signature should be in ink. If an applicant does not sign the declaration for any reason, the Examiner shall not issue a medical certificate but forward the incomplete application to the Aeromedical Certification Division, AAM-300.

EXAMINATION TECHNIQUES AND CRITERIA FOR QUALIFICATION

The following is how the AME and FAA will consider certain medical conditions. This information is also extracted from the *Guide for Aviation Medical Examiners* and covers the more common conditions only. Further elaboration or expectations for conditions not listed should be obtained from your AME. Essentially, the examination portion of your application is documented on the back of Form 8500-8; this is where the AME notes findings and disposition.

The Statement of Demonstrated Ability (SODA) is valid for an indefinite period or until an adverse change occurs that results in a level of defect worse than that stated on the face of the document. The FAA issues SODAs for certain static defects, not for disqualifying conditions that may be progressive. The extent of the functional loss that has been cleared by the FAA is stated on the SODA, and if the AME finds the condition has become worse, a medical certificate should not be issued even if the applicant is otherwise qualified. Conditions listed are for first and second class; these conditions are essentially the same (except first class needs an ECG). Third-class standards are less stringent and can be obtained from your AME.

The following are extracted from the examination section of the AME guide and follow the order found on Form 8500-8.

EAR, NOSE, AND THROAT

• Nose

1. Evidence of severe allergic rhinitis.
2. Malformations that would prevent nasal respiration.
3. Obstruction of sinus ostia, including polyps, that would be likely to result in complete closure.
4. Sinusitis, acute or chronic.

• Ears, general

1. Inner ear: Acute or chronic disease that may disturb equilibrium.
2. Ear drums. Any perforation that has associated pathology is disqualifying for all classes.

• Hearing

The person shall demonstrate acceptable hearing by at least one of the following tests:

1. Demonstrate an ability to hear an average conversational voice in a quiet room, using both ears, at a distance of 6 feet from the examiner, with the back turned to the examiner, or
2. Provide acceptable results of pure tone audiometric testing of unaided hearing acuity according to the following table of worst acceptable thresholds:

Frequency (Hz)	500	1000	2000	3000
Better ear (Db)	35	30	30	40
Poorer ear (Db)	35	50	50	60

If the applicant fails an audiometric test and the conversational voice test had not been administered, the conversational voice test should be performed to determine if the standard applicable to that test can be met. If an applicant is unable to pass either the conversational voice test or the pure tone audiometric test, then an audiometric speech discrimination test should be administered. A passing score is at least 70 percent obtained in one ear at an intensity of no greater than 65 Db.

Applicants who do not meet the auditory standards may be found eligible for a Statement of Demonstrated Ability (SODA).

• Hearing Aids

Under some circumstances, the use of hearing aids may be acceptable. If the applicant is unable to pass any of the above tests without the use of hearing aids, he or she may be tested using hearing aids. If the applicant meets the standard with the use of hearing aids, the certificate may be issued with the following restriction: VALID ONLY WITH USE OF HEARING AMPLIFICATION.

EYE

The following is a partial list of conditions that warrant denial or deferral to the Aeromedical Certification Division. All disqualifying defects are subject to further FAA consideration.

• Eyes, general

1. Hereditary, congenital, or acquired conditions, whether acute or chronic, of either eye or adnexa, that may interfere with visual functions, may progress to that degree, or may be aggravated by flying (i.e., tumors and ptosis obscuring the pupil, acute inflammatory disease of the eyes and lids, cataracts, or orthokeratology).
2. Glaucoma (treated or untreated).

Applicants with many of the foregoing conditions may be found qualified for FAA certification following the receipt and review of specialty evaluations and pertinent medical records. Examples include retinal detachment with surgical correction, open angle glaucoma under adequate control with medication, narrow angle glaucoma following surgical correction, and cataract surgery for applicants for third-class medical certification who have undergone cataract surgery with or without lens(es) implant.

- Distant visual acuity, for First and Second Class of 20/20 or better in each eye separately, with or without corrective lenses. If corrective lenses (spectacles or contact lenses) are necessary for 20/20 vision, the person may be eligible only on the condition that corrective lenses are worn while exercising the privileges of an airman certificate. Each eye will be tested separately, and both eyes together.

An applicant who fails to meet vision standards and has no SODA that covers the extent of the visual acuity defect found on examination may obtain further FAA consideration for grant of an Authorization under the special issuance section of Part 67 for medical certification by submitting a report of an eye evaluation, FAA Form 8500-7, Report of Eye Evaluation, that has been completed by an eye specialist.

- Cataract surgery, with or without lens implant(s), should be deferred issuance of a certificate and all reports should be submitted to the Aeromedical Certification Division, AAM-300, for further consideration.

- Sunglasses

Airmen should be encouraged to use sunglasses in bright daylight but must be cautioned that, under conditions of low illumination, they may compromise vision. Photosensitive lenses are unsuitable for aviation purposes because they respond to changes in light intensity too slowly. The so called "blue blockers" may not be suitable since they block the blue light used in many current panel displays. Polarized sunglasses are unacceptable if the windscreen is also polarized.

- Refractive Surgery: An applicant who has been treated with refractive surgery may be issued a medical certificate by the Examiner if the applicant meets the visual acuity standards and the Report of Eye Evaluation indicates that healing is complete, visual acuity remains stable, and the applicant does not suffer from significant glare intolerance.

- Near vision for First and Second class of 20/40 or better, Snellen equivalent, at 16 inches in each eye separately, with or without corrective lenses. If age 50 or older, near vision of 20/40 or better, Snellen equivalent, at both 16 inches and 32 inches in each eye separately, with or without corrective lenses.

- Bifocal contact lenses or contact lenses that correct for near and/or intermediate vision only are not considered acceptable.

- The use of a contact lens in one eye for distant visual acuity and another in the other eye for near or intermediate visual acuity is not acceptable.

- Color Vision: Ability to perceive those colors necessary for the safe performance of airman duties. An applicant does not meet the color vision standard if testing reveals [partial list of tests]:

1. Seven or more errors on plates 1–15 of the AOC (1965 edition) pseudoisochromatic plates.
2. AOC-HRR (second edition): Any error in test plates 7–11.
3. Seven or more errors on plates 1–15 of Dvorine pseudoisochromatic plates (second edition, 15 plates).
4. Any errors in the six plates of the Titmus Vision Tester.
5. Farnsworth lantern test: An average of more than one error per series of nine color pairs in series 2 and 3.

- Certificate Limitation: If an applicant fails to meet the color vision standard as interpreted above but is otherwise qualified, the Examiner may issue a medical certificate bearing the limitation: NOT VALID FOR NIGHT FLYING OR BY COLOR SIGNAL CONTROL.

- Special Issuance of color deficiency: An applicant who holds a medical certificate bearing a color vision limitation may request reevaluation or a SODA under the special issuance section of Part 67. This request should be in writing and should be directed to the Aeromedical Certification Division, AAM-300. If the applicant can perform the color vision tasks, the FAA will issue a medical certificate without limitation with a SODA. Demonstrating the ability to perform color vision tasks appropriate to the certificate applied for may entail a medical flight test or a signal light test. If a signal light test or medical flight test is required, the FAA will authorize the test. The signal light test may be given at any time during flight training. The medical flight test is most often required when an airman with borderline color vision wishes to upgrade a medical certificate.

- X-Chrom Lens: This lens is not acceptable to the FAA as a means for correcting a pilot's color vision deficiencies.

- Yarn Test: Yarn tests are not acceptable methods of testing for the FAA medical certificate.

- Glaucoma: The Examiner should deny or defer issuance of a medical certificate to an applicant if there is a loss of visual fields, a significant change in visual acuity, a diagnosis of or treatment for glaucoma, or intraocular hypertension. The FAA may grant an Authorization under the special issuance section of Part 67 on an individual basis. The Examiner can facilitate FAA review by obtaining a report of Ophthalmological Evaluation for Glaucoma (FAA Form 8500-14) from a treating or evaluating ophthalmologist.

CARDIOPULMONARY

The following is a partial list of conditions that warrant denial or deferral to the Aeromedical Certification Division. All disqualifying defects are subject to further FAA consideration.

- Lungs and chest

1. The breast examination is performed only at the applicant's option or if indicated by specific history or physical findings.
2. Emphysema, if of sufficient degree to be symptomatic.
3. Chronic obstructive pulmonary disease (COPD).
4. Infectious disease of the lungs, pleura, or mediastinum.
5. Pneumonectomy.
6. Acute fibrinous pleurisy.
7. Spontaneous pneumothorax, until resolved as demonstrated by x ray, and until it is determined that no condition that would be likely to cause recurrence is present.
8. Pneumothorax which is recurrent.
9. Asthma: Except for a history of mild or seasonal asthmatic symptoms, the Examiner should defer issuance for further evaluation and decision. If there is an established diagnosis of moderate or severe asthma, the FAA will usually ask for a report of evaluation by a medical specialist that includes the extent of the disease, medications required, and appropriate pulmonary function studies. Each case is evaluated on an individual basis and, if the FAA finds that an applicant is qualified, a certificate is issued. It may bear certain restrictions and special followup evaluations may be required. When the applicant has asthma that requires use of medication, a report from the treating physician is necessary.

- Heart

1. Myocardial infarction, angina pectoris, or other evidence of coronary heart disease.

2. Permanent cardiac pacemaker implantation.
3. Heart replacement.
4. Valve replacement.
5. Valvular disease of the heart and cardiac valve replacement will be evaluated.
6. Arrhythmia will be evaluated. Arrhythmias caused by organic heart disease and functional arrhythmias, other than sinus arrhythmia or occasional ventricular or atrial ectopic beats, are disqualifying.
7. Congenital heart disease accompanied by cardiac enlargement, ECG abnormality, or evidence of inadequate oxygenation.
8. Pericarditis, endocarditis, or myocarditis.
9. When cardiac arrhythmia, murmur or enlargement, or other evidence of cardiovascular abnormality is found, issuance is deferred. If the applicant wishes further consideration, a consultation will be required "preferably" from a specialist in internal medicine or cardiology. It must include a narrative report of evaluation and be accompanied by an electrocardiogram with report and appropriate laboratory test results which may include, as appropriate, 24-hour Holtor monitoring, thyroid function studies, echocardiography, and an assessment of coronary artery status.

• Vascular system

1. Aneurysm or arteriovenous fistula.
2. Blood and blood-forming tissue disease: a. Anemia; b. Hemophilia; c. Leukemia.
3. Arteriosclerotic vascular disease with evidence of circulatory obstruction.
4. Syncope, not satisfactorily explained or recurrent.

The Examiner should keep in mind some of the special cardiopulmonary demands of flight. Heart rates at take-off and landing sometimes approach age-related maximums. High G-forces of aerobatics or agricultural flying may stress both systems considerably. Degenerative changes are often insidious and may produce subtle performance decrements that may require special investigative techniques.

• Blood Pressure: Measurement of blood pressure is an essential part of the FAA medical certification examination. The average blood pressure while sitting should not exceed 155 mm mercury systolic and 95 mm mercury diastolic maximum pressure for all classes. A medical assessment is specified for all applicants who need or use antihypertensive medication to control blood pressure.

1. An applicant whose pressures are within the above limits, who has not used antihypertensives for 30 days, and who is otherwise qualified should be issued a medical certificate by the Examiner.
2. An applicant whose blood pressure is slightly elevated beyond the FAA specified limits may, at the Examiner's discretion, have a series of three morning and evening blood pressure readings over a 7-day period. If the indication of hypertension remains, even if it is mild or intermittent, the Examiner should defer certification and forward the application to the Aeromedical Certification Division, AAM-300, with a note of explanation.

The Examiner must defer issuance of a medical certificate to any applicant whose hypertension has not been evaluated, who uses unacceptable medications, whose medical status is unclear, whose hypertension is uncontrolled, who manifests significant adverse effects of medication, or whose certification has previously been specifically reserved to the FAA.

• Initial Evaluation for Hypertensives under Treatment

The Examiner may issue first-, second-, or third-class medical certificates to otherwise qualified airmen whose hypertension is adequately controlled with acceptable medications without significant adverse effects. In such cases, the Examiner shall: Conduct an evaluation or, at the applicant's option, review the report of a current (within preceding 6 months) cardiovascular evaluation by the applicant's attending physician. This evaluation must include pertinent personal and family medical history, including an assessment of the risk factors for coronary heart disease, a clinical examination including at least three blood pressure readings, a resting ECG, and a report of fasting plasma glucose, cholesterol (LDL/HDL), triglycerides, potassium, and creatinine levels. A maximal electrocardiographic exercise stress test will be accomplished if it is indicated by history or clinical findings. Specific mention must be made of the medications used, their dosage, and the presence, absence, or history of adverse effects.

• Blood Pressure Medications acceptable to the FAA for treatment of hypertension in airmen include all Food and Drug Administration (FDA) approved diuretics, alpha-adrenergic blocking agents, beta-adrenergic blocking agents, calcium channel blocking agents, angiotension converting enzyme (ACE inhibitors) agents, and direct vasodilators. Centrally acting agents (such as, reserpine, guanethidine, guanadrel, guanabenz, and methyldopa) are not usually acceptable to the FAA. Dosage levels should be the minimum to obtain optimal clinical control and should not be modified to influence the certification decision.

ECG

A person applying for first-class medical certification must demonstrate an absence of myocardial infarction and other clinically significant abnormalities on electrocardiographic examination: At the first application after reaching the 35th birthday; and on an annual basis after reaching the 40th birthday. An ECG will satisfy a requirement of paragraph (b) of this section if it is dated no earlier than 60 days before the date of the application it is to accompany and was performed and transmitted according to acceptable standards and techniques.

• The following is a partial list of conditions that warrant denial or deferral to the Aeromedical Certification Division. All disqualifying defects are subject to further FAA consideration.

A. Arrhythmias, except sinus arrhythmia and occasional atrial or ventricular ectopic beats.
B. Conduction defects such as:
   1. Second degree or complete heart block.
   2. Left bundle branch block.
   3. Acquired right bundle branch block.
C. Other significant findings such as unequivocal ECG evidence of:
   1. Myocardial infarction.
   2. Coronary heart disease.
   3. Ventricular strain.
   4. Ventricular hypertrophy.

• Coronary Heart Disease

Some individuals with a history of myocardial infarction, angina pectoris, cardiac valve replacement, permanent cardiac pacemaker implantation, heart replacement, or coronary heart disease that has required treatment (including coronary artery bypass, coronary angioplasty, or other revascularization procedures; such as, stenting and endarterectomy) or, if untreated, that has been symptomatic or clinically significant may be granted limited certificates through the special issuance section of Part 67 which specifies that an established medical history or clinical diagnosis of the above conditions is cause for denial no matter how remote or whether the applicant is currently symptomatic. It is only through consideration under the special issuance section of Part 67 that the individual may be certified. An Examiner should not issue a certificate to an applicant with such a history unless specifically authorized to do so by the FAA. An applicant's chances for a favorable decision through the special issuance section of Part 67 depend upon many factors as evaluated by medical specialists who advise the FAA. Flight Standards specialists are consulted in situations in which functional limitations must be considered in the interest of aviation safety.

Applicants for first-, second-, or third-class certificates who have had myocardial infarctions, episodes of angina pectoris, cardiac valve replacement, permanent cardiac pacemaker implantation, or who have undergone coronary artery bypass surgery or angioplasty may be considered for Authorization for a Special Issuance of a Medical Certificate (Authorization) after 6 months have elapsed since the event or the surgery. This 6-month period is to allow for stabilization and recovery.

Applicants for any class of certificate who have a history of coronary heart disease must provide the FAA with complete pertinent hospital and other medical records, including admission and discharge summaries, daily progress notes, copies of all electrocardiograms, reports of other diagnostic and treatment procedures, laboratory reports, and outpatient progress notes. Records are required for nonsurgical admissions as well as for surgical admissions.

Authorization for Special Issuance of a Medical Certificate for functionally limited second-class or unlimited third-class certificates may be granted by the FAA in accordance with the following guidance:

(1) A 6-month, or longer as necessary, recovery period shall elapse after the infarction, angina, bypass surgery, or angioplasty to ensure recovery and stability.

(2) As a minimum, a current cardiovascular evaluation, preferably by a specialist in cardiology or internal medicine, shall be obtained. This evaluation must include an assessment of personal and family medical history, a clinical cardiac examination and general physical examination, blood lipid profile, a plasma glucose level, and a maximal electrocardiographic exercise stress test. The evaluation must also include an assessment and statement regarding the applicant's medications, functional capacity, modifiable cardiovascular risk factors, motivation for any necessary change, and prognosis for incapacitation during the certification period. Normally, an applicant will be expected to demonstrate a minimum functional capacity equivalent to completion of stage 3 of the standard Bruce electrocardiographic exercise stress test protocol.

(3) Radionuclide studies may be required if clinically indicated or if the maximal electrocardiographic exercise stress test is equivocal, positive for ischemia, or demonstrates ventricular dysfunction or other significant abnormalities. Either stress MUGA studies, first pass technetium scans, stress echocardiography, Thallium 201 exercise/rest scans, radionuclide

studies, or a combination thereof may be required as appropriate for the individual applicant and recommended by the attending physician or required by the FAA.

(4) All stress testing, including radionuclide studies, must be maximal or symptom-limited. All maximal electrocardiographic exercise stress test tracings, actual scans, and blood pressure/pulse recordings must be submitted.

(5) Cardiac catheterization with coronary angiography will not normally be required for issuance of third-class medical certificates after myocardial infarction, angina pectoris, coronary artery bypass surgery, or coronary angioplasty. If cardiac catheterization and angiography have been accomplished, all reports and films shall be made available for review by the FAA if requested.

(6) If the required evaluation reveals no evidence of ischemia or cardiac dysfunction and the remainder of the examination is favorable, including the absence of significant risk factors, a third-class certificate may be issued by the FAA. Applicants found qualified shall be required to provide cardiovascular evaluations, including a maximal electrocardiographic exercise stress test at least at 12-month intervals as a condition for future certification. If indicated, radionuclide studies and/or other studies may be required.

a. Authorization for Special Issuance of a Medical Certificate for first- and functionally unlimited second-class certificates may be granted by the FAA provided the requirements as outlined above for third-class applicants are met, except that post-event coronary angiography will normally be required. Continued certification of airmen issued certificates in accordance with this paragraph are conditioned on cardiovascular evaluations, including a maximal electrocardiographic exercise stress test at 6-month intervals, plus radionuclide studies at 24-month intervals, unless otherwise indicated or required by the FAA.

b. Consideration for the issuance of functionally limited second-class certificates (e.g., "Not Valid for Carrying Passengers for Compensation or Hire," etc.). Authorization for Special Issuance of a Medical Certificate may be granted by the FAA provided the requirements as outlined are met. Usually post-event coronary angiography is not required unless specifically indicated by the findings.

For all classes, certification decisions will be based on the applicant's medical history and current clinical findings. First- or unlimited second-class certification is unlikely unless the information is highly favorable to the applicant. Evidence of extensive multi-vessel disease, impaired cardiac functioning, precarious coronary circulation, etc., will preclude certification. Before an applicant undergoes coronary angiography, it is recommended that all records and the report of a current cardiovascular evaluation, including a maximal electrocardiographic exercise stress test, be submitted to the FAA for preliminary review. Based upon this information, it may be possible to advise an applicant of the likelihood of favorable consideration.

- Heart Murmur: When the Examiner discovers a heart murmur during the course of conducting a routine FAA examination, it should be noted whether it is functional or organic and if a special examination is needed.

- Surgery: The presence of an aneurysm or obstruction of a major vessel of the body is disqualifying for medical certification of any class. Following successful surgical intervention and correction, the applicant may ask for FAA consideration. The FAA recommends that the applicant recover for at least 3-6 months. The likelihood of certification is enhanced in situations in which all medications have been discontinued and a current evaluation reveals no evidence of cardiovascular or renal disease.

A history of coronary artery bypass surgery is disqualifying for certification. Such surgery does not negate a past history of coronary heart disease. For details, see paragraph 2 of this section. The presence of permanent cardiac pacemakers and artificial heart valves is also disqualifying for certification. The FAA will consider an Authorization for a Special Issuance of a Medical Certificate (Authorization) for all the above conditions. Applicants seeking further FAA consideration should be prepared to submit all past records and a report of a complete current cardiovascular evaluation in accordance with FAA specifications.

- Vascular Disease: Arteriosclerotic disease, when mild, may present no impediment to medical certification. At some point in the natural course of this disease process, the nature and severity of related symptoms or the potential for incapacitation may preclude continued certification. This is certainly true by the time surgical intervention is contemplated. Following surgery (such as an endarterectomy), the FAA will consider an Authorization under the special issuance section of Part 67 unless significant uncorrected disease remains. However, in addition to recovery from surgery and demonstration that the disease is not severe, these individuals must also show that there are no neurological deficits or signs of other cardiovascular disease, especially of the coronary arteries.

The applicant who has a history of pulmonary embolus without sequelae or need for medication may be certified. Often, such individuals are placed upon prophylactic or maintenance anticoagulant therapy such as warfarin.

Use of any anticoagulant medication is disqualifying but can be considered for an Authorization under the special issuance section of Part 67. When medical management results in a clinical status wherein medication is no longer a requirement, prospects for a favorable certification decision by the FAA are much improved.

ABDOMEN AND VISCERA AND ANUS

• The following is a partial list of conditions that warrant initial denial.

1. Cholelithiasis. (Gallstones)
2. Cirrhosis.
3. Hepatitis, acute; or chronic with impaired liver function.
4. Ventral or hiatal hernia, if symptomatic; or any hernia likely to incarcer-ate or strangulate.
5. Malignancy.

• Peptic ulcer. Following is a special procedure for ulcer. An applicant with a history of an active ulcer within the past 3 months or a bleeding ulcer within the past 6 months must provide evidence that the ulcer is healed if consideration for medical certification is desired. Evidence of healing must be verified by a report from the attending physician that includes the fol-lowing information:
    Confirmation that the applicant is free of symptoms.
    Radiographic or endoscopic evidence that the ulcer has healed.
    Type, dosage, and frequency of medication used.

Under favorable circumstances, the FAA may issue a certificate with special requirements. For example, an applicant with a history of bleeding ulcer may be required to have the physician submit followup reports every 6 months for 1 year following initial certification. The prophylactic use of medications including simple antacids, H-2 inhibitors or blockers, and/or sucralfates may not be disqualifying. An applicant with a history of gastric resection for ulcer may be favorably considered if free of sequelae.

• Regional enteritis. The episodic occurrence of symptoms and the need for medications and the type of medications used for treatment of regional enteritis are of concern to the FAA. Six months after surgery, however, the applicant's eligibility for medical certification could be established upon written evidence from the surgeon that recovery is complete. An applicant after a colectomy with an ileostomy or a colostomy may also receive FAA consideration. A report is necessary to confirm that the applicant has fully recovered from the surgery and is completely asymptomatic.

GENITO-URINARY SYSTEM

The following is a partial list of conditions that warrant potential denial. All disqualifying defects are subject to further FAA consideration.

1. Calculus (stone): renal, ureteral, or vesical.
2. Tumors or malignancies, including prostatic carcinoma, require further evaluation.
3. Retained stones are disqualifying for issuance of a medical certificate. Complete studies to determine the possible etiology and prognosis are essential to favorable FAA consideration. Determining factors include site and location of the stones, complications such as compromise in renal function, repeated bouts of kidney infection, and need for therapy. Any underlying disease will be considered. The likelihood of sudden incapacitating symptoms is of primary concern.
4. Glycosuria (sugar in the urine) requires special evaluation.
5. Renal dialysis and transplant are cause for denial. FAA certification may be possible after complete recovery from surgery and in limited circumstances involving dialysis.

- Urinalysis: No established medical history or clinical diagnosis of diabetes mellitus that requires insulin or any other hypoglycemic drug for control. Glycosuria or proteinuria is cause for deferral of medical certificate issuance until additional studies determine the status of the endocrine and/or urinary systems. If the glycosuria has been determined not to be due to carbohydrate intolerance, the Examiner may issue the certificate. Trace or 1+ proteinuria in the absence of a history of renal disease is not cause for denial.

- Pregnancy under normal circumstances is not disqualifying. It is recommended that the applicant's obstetrician be made aware of all aviation activities so that the obstetrician can properly advise the applicant. The Examiner may wish to counsel applicants concerning piloting aircraft during the third trimester, and the proper use of lap belt and shoulder harness warrants discussion.

SPINE, OTHER MUSCULOSKELETAL

The following are subject to further testing:

1. Symptomatic herniation of intervertebral disc.
2. Other disturbances of musculoskeletal function.
3. Arthritis, if it is symptomatic or requires medication (other than small

doses of nonprescription anti-inflammatory agents), is disqualifying un-less the applicant holds a letter from the FAA specifically authorizing the Examiner to issue the certificate when the applicant is found otherwise qualified. Although the use of many medications on a continuing basis ordinarily contraindicates the performance of pilot duties, under certain circumstances, certification is possible for an applicant who is taking as-pirin, ibuprofen, naproxen, or similar nonsteroidal anti-inflammatory drugs (NSAID). If the applicant presents evidence documenting that the un-derlying condition for which the medicine is being taken is not in itself disabling and the applicant has been on therapy (NSAID) long enough to have established that the medication is well tolerated and has not pro-duced adverse side effects, the Examiner may issue a certificate.

4. A history of intervertebral disc surgery is not disqualifying. If the appli-cant is asymptomatic, has completely recovered from surgery, is taking no medication, and has suffered no neurological deficit, the Examiner should confirm these facts in a brief statement under Item 60 of FAA Form 8500-8 or in a letter attached to the application. The Examiner may then issue any class of medical certificate, providing that the individual meets all the medical standards for that class.

NEUROLOGICAL

The following is a partial list of conditions that warrant potential denial. All disqualifying defects are subject to further FAA consideration.

• An established history of any of the following conditions is disqualifying for medical certification:

1. Epilepsy.
2. Transient loss of nervous system function(s) without satisfactory med-ical explanation of the cause; e.g., transient global amnesia.
3. A disturbance of consciousness without satisfactory medical explana-tion of the cause; e.g., unexplained syncope, single seizure.

An applicant who has a history of epilepsy, a disturbance of consciousness without satisfactory medical explanation of the cause, or a transient loss of control of nervous system function(s) without satisfactory medical explana-tion of the cause must be denied or deferred by the Examiner. Infrequently, the FAA has granted an Authorization under the special issuance section of Part 67 when a seizure disorder was present in childhood but the individual has been seizure-free for a number of years. Factors that would be considered in determining eligibility in such cases would be age at onset, nature and frequency of seizures, precipitating causes, and duration of stability without medication. Followup evaluations are usually necessary to confirm continued stability of an individual's condition if an Authorization is granted under the special issuance section of Part 67.

Applicants who have a history of an unexplained disturbance of consciousness may also be granted an Authorization under the special issuance section of Part 67, but usually only after a prolonged period without recurrent episodes.

4. A history or the presence of the following condition precludes issuance of a medical certificate: Head trauma associated with unconsciousness or disorientation of more than 1 hour following injury.
   a. Focal neurologic deficit.
   b. Depressed skull fracture.
   c. Post-traumatic headache.
   d. Subdural or epidural hematoma.

Complete neurological evaluation with appropriate laboratory and imaging studies will be required to determine an applicant's eligibility. A period of stabilization will usually be required to confirm that an applicant has adequately recovered from any of the above conditions before he or she is considered for medical certification.

5. Headache: a. Migraine, b. Migraine equivalent, c. Cluster headache, d. Chronic tension headache.

6. Vertigo or disequilibrium. Meniere's disease and acute peripheral vestibulopathy. Numerous conditions may affect equilibrium, resulting in acute incapacitation or varying degrees of chronic recurring spatial disorientation. Prophylactic use of medications also may affect pilot performance. In most instances, further neurological evaluation will be required to determine eligibility for medical certification; therefore, issuance of a medical certificate should be deferred.

7. Cerebrovascular disease (including the brain stem).
   a. Transient ischemic attack (TIA).
   b. Brain infarction.
   c. Intracerebral or subarachnoid hemorrhage.
   d. Intracranial aneurysm or arteriovenous malformation.

Complete neurological evaluations supplemented with appropriate laboratory and imaging studies are required of applicants with the above conditions. Cerebral arteriography may be necessary for review in cases of subarachnoid hemorrhage.

8. Intracranial tumor. A variety of intracranial tumors, both malignant and benign, are capable of causing incapacitation directly by neurologic deficit or indirectly through recurrent symptomatology. Potential neurologic deficits include weakness, loss of sensation, ataxia, visual deficit, or mental impairment. Recurrent symptomatology may interfere with flight performance through mechanisms such as seizure, headaches, vertigo, visual disturbances, or confusion. A history or diagnosis of an intracranial tumor necessitates a complete neurological evaluation with appropriate laboratory and imaging studies before a determination of eligibility for medical certification can be established. An applicant with a history of benign supratentorial tumors may be considered favorably for medical certification by the FAA and returned to flying status after a minimum satisfactory convalescence of 1 year.

9. Spasticity, weakness, or paralysis of the extremities. Conditions that are stable and nonprogressive may be considered for medical certification. In addition to hospital records, the information necessary for determining eligibility for medical certification includes the medical history, etiology of the neurological condition, degree of involvement, period of stability, and total current health and neurological status of the individual. Neurological consultation, including appropriate laboratory and imaging studies, will be required. The Examiner should defer issuance of a medical certificate and forward all records to the Aeromedical Certification Division, AAM-300.

10. Multiple sclerosis.

11. Infections of the nervous system: a. Meningitis, b. AIDS. Many different types of infection of the nervous system exist, and postinfectious complications and degree of recovery may differ widely. The most significant factors to be considered include the possibility of a seizure disorder or mental impairment. A complete neurological evaluation with appropriate laboratory and imaging studies will be required to determine eligibility for medical certification.

Because of the variability and unpredictability of involvement and course of the above conditions, the FAA must consider each applicant's case to determine eligibility for medical certification. Factors used in determining eligibility will include the medical history, neurological involvement and persisting deficit, period of stability without symptoms, type and dosage of medications used, and general health. A neurological and/or general medical consultation will be necessary in most instances. The Examiner should defer issuance of a medical certificate and forward all medical records to the Aeromedical Certification Division.

Considerable variability exists in the severity of involvement, rate of progression, and treatment of the above conditions. A complete neurological evaluation with appropriate laboratory and imaging studies, including information specifically on the above factors, will be necessary for determination of eligibility for medical certification.

Conditions that have a poor prognosis will likely be denied. The applicant should not be encouraged to pursue medical certification.

PSYCHIATRIC

• General Considerations of psychiatric disorder

It must be pointed out that considerations for safety, which in the "mental" area are related to a compromise of judgment and emotional control or to diminished mental capacity with loss of behavioral control, are not the same as concerns for emotional health in everyday life. Some problems may have only a slight impact on an individual's overall capacities and the quality of life but may nevertheless have a great impact on safety. Conversely, many emotional problems that are of therapeutic and clinical concern have no impact on safety.

The reasons that an applicant has seen a mental health professional need to be revealed, but may be found not to have significance for medical certification. For instance, growth and adjustment problems requiring psychotherapy are usually not considered significant for safety when there have been no vocational disruptions and medications have not been used. This might include marital counseling or psychotherapy for identity problems or issues of growth and personal fulfillment. A history of brief situational problems secondary to such life events as marital disruption, business problems, and the death of loved ones may likewise not be significant. Also, sexual behavior that does not reflect upon overall judgment and self control is not a concern for safety.

● Denials

The FAA has concluded that certain psychiatric conditions are such that their presence or a past history of their presence is sufficient to suggest a significant potential threat to safety. It is, therefore, incumbent upon the Examiner to be aware of any indications of these conditions currently, or in the past, and to deny or defer issuance of the medical certificate to an applicant who has a history of these conditions. An applicant who has a current diagnosis or history of these conditions (listed below) may request the FAA to grant an Authorization under the special issuance section of Part 67 and, based upon individual considerations, the FAA may grant such an issuance.

1. The category of personality disorder severe enough to have repeatedly manifested itself by overt acts refers to diagnosed personality disorders that involve what is called "acting out" behavior. These personality problems relate to poor social judgment, impulsivity, and disregard or antagonism toward authority, especially rules and regulations. A history of long-standing behavioral problems, whether major (criminal) or relatively minor (truancy, military misbehavior, petty criminal and civil indiscretions, and social instability), usually occurs with these disorders. Driving infractions and previous failures to follow aviation regulations are critical examples of these acts.

2. The category of psychosis includes schizophrenia and some bipolar and major depression, as well as some other rarer conditions. In addition, some conditions such as schizotypal and borderline personality disorders that include psychotic symptoms at some time in their course may also be disqualifying.

3. A bipolar disorder may not reach the level of psychosis but can be so disruptive of judgment and functioning (especially mania) so as to interfere with aviation safety. All applicants with such a diagnosis must be denied or deferred. However, a number of these applicants, so diagnosed, may be favorably considered for an Authorization when the symptoms do not constitute a threat to safe aviation operations.

4. Certain personality disorders and other mental disorders that include conditions of limited duration and/or widely varying severity may be disqualifying. Under this category, the FAA is especially concerned with significant depressive episodes requiring treatment, even outpatient therapy. If these episodes have been severe enough to cause some disruption of vocational or educational activity, or if they have required

medication or involved suicidal ideation, the application should be deferred or denied issuance. Some personality disorders and situational dysphorias may be considered disqualifying for a limited time. These include such conditions as gross immaturity and some personality disorders not involving or manifested by overt acts. Although they may be rare in occurrence, severe anxiety problems, especially anxiety and phobias associated with some aspect of flying, are considered significant. Organic mental disorders that cause a cognitive defect, even if the applicant is not psychotic, are considered disqualifying whether they are due to trauma, toxic exposure, or arteriosclerotic or other degenerative changes.

5. Substance dependence refers to the use of substances of dependence, which include alcohol and other drugs (i.e., PCP, sedatives and hypnotics, anxiolytics, marijuana, cocaine, opioids, amphetamines, hallucinogens, and other psychoactive drugs or chemicals). Substance dependence is defined and specified as a disqualifying medical condition. It is disqualifying unless there is clinical evidence, satisfactory to the Federal Air Surgeon, of recovery, including sustained total abstinence from the substance for not less than the preceding 2 years.

Substance dependence is evidenced by one or more of the following: Increased tolerance, manifestation of withdrawal symptoms; impaired control of use; or continued use despite damage to physical health or impairment of social, personal, or occupational functioning. Substance dependence is accompanied by various deleterious effects on physical health as well as personal or social functioning. There are many other indicators of substance dependence in the history and physical examination. Treatment for substance dependence–related problems, arrests, including charges of driving under the influence of drugs or alcohol, and vocational or marital disruption related to drugs or alcohol consumption are important indicators. Alcohol on the breath at the time of a routine physical examination should arouse a high index of suspicion. Consumption of drugs or alcohol sufficient to cause liver damage is an indication of the presence of alcoholism.

6. Substance abuse includes the use of the above substances under any one of the following conditions:

   a. Use of a substance in the last 2 years in which the use was physically hazardous (e.g., DUI or DWI) if there has been at any other time an instance of the use of a substance also in a situation in which the use was physically hazardous;

   b. If a person has received a verified positive drug test result under an anti-drug program of the Department of Transportation or one of its administrations; or

c. The Federal Air Surgeon finds that an applicant's misuse of a substance makes him or her unable to safely perform the duties or exercise the privileges of the airman certificate applied for or held, or that may reasonably be expected, for the maximum duration of the airman medical certificate applied for or held, to make the applicant unable to perform those duties or exercise those privileges.

Substance dependence and substance abuse are specified as disqualifying medical conditions.

7. The use of a psychotropic drug is considered disqualifying. This includes all sedatives, tranquilizers, antipsychotic drugs, antidepressant drugs (including SSRI's), analeptics, anxiolytics, and hallucinogens. The Examiner should defer issuance and forward the medical records to the Aeromedical Certification Division.

GENERAL SYSTEMIC

• Hypothyroidism. The use of thyroid replacement therapy following Rx of either hyperthyroidism or hypothyroidism is not disqualifying if the applicant appears clinically euthyroid pending receipt of confirmatory laboratory tests. Otherwise the application should be deferred and all reports forwarded with the application to the Aeromedical Certification Division, for a determination.

• Diabetes Mellitus. A blood glucose determination is not a routine part of the FAA medical evaluation for any class of medical certificate. However, the examination does include a routine urinalysis. A medical history or clinical diagnosis of diabetes mellitus may be considered previously established when the diagnosis has been or clearly could be made because of supporting laboratory findings and/or clinical signs and symptoms. When an applicant with a history of diabetes is examined for the first time, the Examiner should explain the procedures involved and assist in obtaining prior records and current special testing. Applicants with a diagnosis of diabetes mellitus controlled by diet alone are considered eligible for all classes of medical certificates under the medical standards provided they have no evidence of associated disqualifying cardiovascular, neurological, renal, or ophthalmological disease. Specialized examinations need not be performed unless indicated by history or clinical findings. The Examiner should document these determinations on FAA Form 8500-8.

Applicants with a diagnosis of diabetes mellitus controlled by use of an oral hypoglycemic medication may be considered by the FAA for Special Issuance of a Medical Certificate (Authorization). Following initiation of oral medication treatment, a 60 day period must elapse prior to certification to assure stabilization, adequate control, and the absence of side effects or complications from the medication.

Initial certification decisions shall not be made by the Examiner. These cases will be deferred to the Aeromedical Certification Division, AAM-300. Examiners may be delegated authority to make subsequent certification decisions, subject to further Aeromedical Certification Division review and consideration.

The initial determination of eligibility will be made on the basis of a report from the treating physician. For favorable consideration, the report must contain a statement regarding the medication used, dosage, the absence or presence of side effects and clinically significant hypoglycemic episodes, and an indication of satisfactory control of the diabetes. The results of an A1C hemoglobin determination within the past 30 days must be included. Note must also be made of the absence or presence of cardiovascular, neurological, renal, and/or ophthalmological disease. The presence of one or more of these associated diseases shall not be, per se, disqualifying, but the disease(s) shall be carefully evaluated to determine any added risk to aviation safety.

Recertification decisions will also be made on the basis of reports from the treating physician. The contents of the report must contain the same information required for initial certification and specifically reference the presence or absence of satisfactory control, any change in the dosage or type of oral hypoglycemic drug, and the presence or absence of complications or side effects from the medication. In the event of an adverse change in the applicant's diabetic status (poor control or complications or side effects from the medication), or the appearance of an associated systemic disease, an Examiner who has been given the authority to issue a certificate pending further review and consideration by the Aeromedical Certification Division shall defer certification to the Aeromedical Certification Division, AAM-300. If, upon further review, it is decided that recertification is appropriate, the Examiner may again be given the authority to issue certificates (subject to the Aeromedical Certification Division, review and consideration) based on data provided by the treating physician, including such information as may be required to assess the associated medical condition(s).

As a minimum, followup evaluations by the treating physician of the applicant's diabetic status shall be required at 6 months for first-class certification, and at 1 year for second- and third-class certification.

Airmen who are diabetics should be counseled by Examiners regarding the significance of their disease and its possible complications. They should be informed of the potential for hypoglycemic reactions and cautioned to remain under close medical surveillance by their treating physicians. They should also be advised that should their oral medications be changed or dosages modified they should not perform airman duties until the treating physician has concluded that their conditions are under control and present no hazard to aviation safety.

Note: The FAA will consider certification for third class those pilots with insulin-treated diabetes. See Appendix III. The following information from the *Guide for Aviation Medical Examiners* discusses the items on the back of Form 8500-8; these concern the actions the AME should take after the examination.

ITEM 60. COMMENTS ON HISTORY AND FINDINGS

In addition to comments on positive historical or examination findings, this item gives the Examiner an opportunity to report observations and/or findings that are not asked for in other items on the application form. Concern about the applicant's behavior, abnormal situations arising during the conduct of tests, unusual findings, unreported history, and other information thought germane to aviation safety should be reported under Item 60 or on a separate sheet of paper.

If possible, all ancillary reports such as consultations, ECG's, x-ray release forms, and hospital or other treatment records should be attached. If the delay for those items would exceed 14 days, the Examiner should forward all available data to the Aeromedical Certification Division, AAM-300, with a note specifying what additional information is being prepared for submission at a later date.

If there are no significant medical history items or abnormal physical findings, the Examiner should indicate this by checking the appropriate block.

ITEM 62. HAS BEEN ISSUED

The Examiner must check the proper box to indicate if the Medical Certificate, FAA Form 8500-9 (white), or Medical Certificate and Student Pilot Certificate, FAA Form 8420-2 (yellow), has been issued. If neither form has been issued, the Examiner must indicate denial or deferral by checking one of the two lower boxes. If denied, a copy of the Examiner's letter of denial, FAA Form 8500-2, should be attached to the report sent to the Aeromedical Certification Division, AAM-300.

• Issuance

When the Examiner receives all the supplemental information requested and finds that the applicant meets all the FAA medical standards for the class sought, the Examiner should issue a medical certificate.

• Deferral

If upon receipt of the information the Examiner finds there is a need for even more information or there is uncertainty about the significance of the findings, certification should be deferred. The Examiner's concerns should be noted on FAA Form 8500-8 and the application forwarded to the Aeromedical Certification Division, AAM-300, for further consideration.

Appendix III

Certification of Insulin-Treated Diabetes Mellitus (ITDM) Pilots

The following is extracted from the FAA's December 1996 policy change regarding the consideration of diabetic pilots for medical certification. While the policy is self-explanatory, for specific details relative to their own condition, pilots should contact an AME.

Special Issuance of Third-Class Airman Medical Certificates to Insulin-Treated Diabetes Mellitus Airman Applicants

... the Federal Air Surgeon has determined that selected ITDM individuals can be considered for special issuance of an airman medical certificate under the conditions of the evaluation and monitoring protocol with the following restrictions:

(1) ITDM individuals may be issued only a third-class airman medical certificate.
(2) ITDM individuals may exercise only the privileges of a student, recreational, or private pilot certificate.
(3) ITDM individuals are prohibited from operating an aircraft as a required crewmember on any flight outside the airspace of the United States of America.
(4) ITDM individuals are required to be in compliance with the monitoring requirements of the following protocol while exercising the privileges of a third-class airman medical certificate:

I. Initial Evaluation of Individuals with Insulin-Treated Diabetes Mellitus.

A. Individuals with ITDM who have no otherwise disqualifying conditions, especially significant diabetes-related complications such as arteriosclerotic coronary or cerebral disease, retinal disease, or chronic renal failure, will be evaluated for special issuance of a third-class medical certificate if they:

1. Have had no recurrent (two or more) hypoglycemic reactions resulting in a loss of consciousness or seizure within the past 5 years. A period of 1 year of demonstrated stability is required following the first episode of hypoglycemia; and

2. Have had no recurrent hypoglycemic reactions requiring intervention by another party within the past 5 years. A period of 1 year of demonstrated stability is required following the first episode of hypoglycemia; and

3. Have had no recurrent hypoglycemic reactions resulting in impaired cognitive function which occurred without warning symptoms within the past 5 years. A period of 1 year of demonstrated stability is required following the first episode of hypoglycemia.

B. In order to provide an adequate basis for an individual medical determination, the person with ITDM seeking special issuance of a medical certificate must submit the following to:

Federal Aviation Administration
Civil Aeromedical Institute, AAM-310
6500 South MacArthur
Oklahoma City, OK 73125

1. Copies of all medical records concerning the individual's diabetes diagnosis and disease history and copies of all hospital records, if admitted for any diabetes-related cause, including accidents and injuries;

2. Copies of complete reports of any incidents or accidents, particularly involving moving vehicles, whether or not the event resulted in injury or property damage, if due in part or totally to diabetes;

3. Results of a complete medical evaluation by an endocrinologist or other diabetes specialist physician acceptable to the Federal Air Surgeon (hereafter referred to as "specialist"). This report should detail the individual's complete medical history and current medical condition. The report must include a general physical examination and, at a minimum, the following information:

    (a) Two measurements of glycosylated hemoglobin (total A1 or A1C concentration and the laboratory reference normal range), the first at least 90 days prior to the current measurement;

    (b) A detailed report of the individual's insulin dosages (including types) and diet utilized for glucose control;

    (c) Appropriate examinations and tests to detect any peripheral neuropathy or circulatory insufficiency of the extremities;

    (d) Confirmation by an ophthalmologist of the absence of clinically significant eye disease. The eye examination should assess, at a minimum, visual acuity, ocular tension, and presence of lenticular opacities, if any, and include a careful examination of the retina for evidence of any diabetic retinopathy or macular edema. The presence of microaneurysms, exudates, or other findings of background retinopathy, by themselves, are not sufficient grounds for disqualification unless it prevents the subject from meeting visual standards. However, individuals with active proliferative retinopathy or vitreous hemorrhages will not be considered for special issuance of a medical certificate until the condition has stabilized and this has been confirmed by an ophthalmologist; and

4. Verification by a specialist that the individual has been educated in diabetes and its control and has been thoroughly informed of and understands the monitoring and management procedures for the condition and the actions that should be followed if complications of diabetes, including hypoglycemia, should arise. Such verification should also contain the specialist's evaluation as to whether the individual has the ability and willingness to properly monitor and manage his or her diabetes and whether diabetes will adversely affect his or her ability to safely control an aircraft. The presence or absence of recurrent severe hypoglycemia and hypoglycemia unawareness should be noted. (See I.A.1, 2, and 3 above.)

C. The ITDM individual applying for special issuance of a medical certificate should have been receiving appropriate insulin treatment for at least 6 months prior to submitting a request for special issuance of a medical certificate.

D. Special medical flight test. If the Federal Air Surgeon determines that there is need for an ITDM applicant to demonstrate his or her ability to comply with the medical protocol, the Federal Air Surgeon, under the provisions of FAR 67.401, may require a special medical examination and/or medical flight test prior to a determination of the applicant's eligibility for special issuance of a medical certificate.

II. Guidelines for Individuals with ITDM Who Have Been Granted Special Issuance of Airman Medical Certificates.

A. Individuals with ITDM who are granted special issuance of third-class airman medical certificates must:

1. Submit to a medical evaluation by a specialist every 3 months. This evaluation must include a general physical examination and a report of glycosylated hemoglobin (total A1 or A1C) concentration. This evaluation shall also contain an assessment of the individual's continued ability and willingness to monitor and manage properly his or her diabetes and of whether the individual's diabetes or its complications could reasonably be expected to adversely affect his or her ability to safely control an aircraft.

2. Carry and use a digital whole blood glucose measuring device with

memory that is acceptable to the FAA. Provide records of all daily blood glucose measurements for review by the specialist at each 3-month evaluation required above and, if required, to the FAA at any time.

3. Provide to the FAA, on an annual basis, written confirmation by a specialist that the individual's diabetes remains under control and without significant complications and that he or she has demonstrated reasonable accuracy and recordation of his or her blood glucose measurements with the above described device.

4. Provide to the FAA, on an annual basis, confirmation by an ophthalmologist of the absence of clinically significant disease that would prevent the individual from meeting current visual standards.

5. Provide to the FAA, immediately, a written report of any episode of hypoglycemia associated with cognitive impairment, whether or not it resulted in an accident or adverse event.

6. Provide a written report to the FAA, immediately, of involvement in any accidents, including those involving aircraft and motor vehicles, or other significant adverse events, whether or not they are believed related to an episode of hypoglycemia.

7. Provide to the FAA, immediately upon determination by a specialist or other physician, any evidence of loss of diabetes control, significant complications, or inability to manage the diabetes. In such a case, the individual shall cease exercising the privileges of his or her airman certificate until again cleared medically by the FAA.

III. Glucose Management prior to Flight, during Flight, and prior to Landing.

A. Individuals with ITDM shall maintain appropriate medical supplies for glucose management at all times while preparing for flight and while acting as pilot-in-command (or other flightcrew member). At a minimum, such supplies shall include:

1. an FAA-acceptable whole blood digital glucose monitor with memory;

2. supplies needed to obtain adequate blood samples and to measure whole blood glucose; and

3. an amount of rapidly absorbable glucose, in 10 gram (gm) portions, appropriate to the potential duration of the flight.

B. All disposable supplies listed above must be within their expiration dates.

C. The individual with ITDM, acting as pilot-in-command or other flightcrew member, shall establish and document a blood glucose concentration equal to or greater than 100 milligrams/deciliter (mg/dl) but not greater than 300 mg/dl within ½ hour prior to takeoff. During flight, the individual with ITDM shall monitor his or her blood glucose concentration at hourly intervals and within ½ hour prior to landing. If a blood glucose concentration range of 100-300 mg/dl is not maintained, the following action shall be taken:

   1. Prior to flight. The individual with ITDM shall test and record his or her blood glucose concentration within ½ hour prior to takeoff. If blood glucose measures less than 100 mg/dl, the individual shall ingest an appropriate 10 gm glucose snack (minimum 10 gm) and recheck and document blood glucose concentration after ½ hour. This process shall be repeated until blood glucose concentration is in the 100-300 mg/dl range. If blood glucose concentration measures greater than 300 mg/dl, the individual shall follow his or her regimen of blood glucose control, as provided to the FAA by his or her attending physician, until the measurement of blood glucose concentration permits adherence to this protocol.

   2. During flight.

   (a) One hour into the flight, at each successive hour of flight, and within ½ hour prior to landing, the individual shall measure and document his or her blood glucose concentration. Listed below are blood glucose concentration ranges and the actions to be taken when they occur during flight:

      (1) Less than 100 mg/dl: The individual shall ingest a 20 gm glucose snack and recheck and document his or her blood glucose concentration after 1 hour.

      (2) 100–300 mg/dl: The individual may continue his or her flight as planned.

      (3) Greater than 300 mg/dl: The individual shall land as soon as practicable at the nearest suitable airport.

   (b) The individual, as pilot, is responsible for the safety of the flight and must remain cognizant of those factors that are important in its successful completion. Accordingly, in recognition of such elements as adverse weather, turbulence, air traffic control changes, or other variables, the individual may decide that a scheduled, hourly measurement of blood glucose concentration during the flight is of lower priority than the need for full, undivided attention to piloting. In such cases, the individual shall ingest a 10 gm glucose snack. One hour after ingestion of this glucose snack, the individual shall measure and document his or her blood glucose concentration. If the individual is unable to perform the measurement of his or her blood glucose concentration for the second consecutive time, the individual shall ingest a 20 gm glucose snack and shall land as soon as practicable at the nearest suitable airport. The individual, under these circumstances, is not required to measure and document his or her blood glucose concentration within ½ hour prior to landing.

3. Prior to landing. Except as noted above, the individual must measure and document his or her blood glucose concentration within ½ hour prior to landing.

MONITORING AND ACTIONS REQUIRED DURING FLIGHT OPERATIONS

(Extracted from the Federal Air Surgeon's Medical Bulletin for winter 1996)

To ensure safe flight, the insulin-using diabetic airman must carry during flight a whole blood glucose monitor with memory, adequate supplies to obtain blood samples, and an amount of rapidly absorbable glucose, in 10 gm portions, appropriate to the planned duration of the flight. The following actions shall be taken in connection with flight operations:

1. One-half hour prior to flight, he or she must measure the blood glucose concentration. If it is less than 100 mg/dl., the individual must ingest an appropriate (not less than 10 gm) glucose snack and measure the glucose concentration one-half hour later. If the concentration is within 100-300 mg/dl, flight operations may be undertaken. If less than 100, the process must be repeated; if over 300, the flight must be canceled.

2. One hour into the flight, at each successive hour of flight, and within one-half hour prior to landing, the airman shall measure his or her blood glucose concentration. If the concentration is less than 100 mg/dl, a 20 gm glucose snack shall be ingested. If the concentration is 100-300 mg/dl, no action is required. If the concentration is greater than 300 mg/dl, the airman must land at the nearest suitable airport and may not resume flight until the glucose concentration can be maintained in the 100-300 mg/dl range. In respect to determining blood glucose concentrations during flight, the airman must use judgment in deciding whether measuring concentrations or operational demands of the environment (e.g., adverse weather) should take priority. In cases where it is decided that operational demands take priority, the airman must ingest a 10 gm glucose snack and measure his or her blood glucose level 1 hour later. If measurement is not practical at that time, the airman must ingest a 20 gm glucose snack and land at the nearest suitable airport so that a determination of the blood glucose concentration may be made.

3. In addition to the medical assessment, the applicant will be required to demonstrate to a flight instructor or FAA aviation safety inspector the applicant's ability to obtain blood and make a blood glucose determination while safely controlling an aircraft in flight.

Index

FAA regulations concerning specific diseases appear in bold face.